SAMUEL HAHNEMANN

ORGANON
OF
MEDICINE

ORGANON
OF
MEDICINE

By

SAMUEL HAHNEMANN

Sixth Edition
Hahnemann's Own Written Revision

Translated By

WILLIAM BOERICKE, M.D.

B. JAIN PUBLISHERS PVT. LTD.

Price : Rs. 40.00

Reprint Edition 1995

© Copyright with Publishers

Publish   by :
B. Jain Publishers Pvt. LTD.
7, Wazir Pur Printing Press Complex,
Ring Road, Delhi-110 052 (INDIA)

Printed in India by :
J.J. Offset Printers
7, Wazirpur, Delhi-110 052

ISBN 81—7021—085—2
BOOK CODE B-2264

TRANSLATOR'S PREFACE.

The sixth edition of the "Organon" as left by Hahnemann ready for publication, was found to be an interleaved copy of the fifth, the last German Edition, published in 1833. In his eighty-sixth year, while in active practice in Paris, he completed the thorough revision of it by carefully going over paragraph by paragraph, making changes, erasures, annotations and additions.

Hahnemann himself had apprized several friends of the preparation of another edition of his great work as is evident among others from a letter to Bœnninghausen, his most appreciative follower and intimate friend. Writing to him from Paris, he states: "I am at work on the sixth edition of the 'Organon,' to which I devote several hours on Sundays and Thursdays, all the other time being required for treatment of patients who come to my rooms." And to his publisher, Mr. Schaub, in Dusseldorf, he wrote in a letter dated Paris, February 20, 1842: "I have now, after eighteen months of work, finished the sixth edition of my 'Organon,' the most nearly perfect of all." He further expressed the wish to have it printed in the best possible style as regards paper, perfectly new type and in short desired its appearance to be unexceptionally fine as it would most likely be the last. These wishes of the venerable author have been carried out perfectly by the present publishers.

All these annotations, changes, and additions I have carefully translated from the original copy in my possession. Hahnemann made these in his own wonderfully small, clear handwriting, perfectly preserved during all

3

these years and as legible today as when first written. For those extensive parts in which he made no changes whatever, including his long Introduction, I have adopted Dr. Dudgeon's fine translation of the fifth edition, which has the distinction of perfect English with a remarkable, faithful adherence to the peculiar Hahnemannian style and setting.

The following are some of the more important changes noted in this final edition.

In a long footnote to Paragraph 11 he gives a consideration of the important question: What is Dynamic Influence—Dynamis—and in Paragraphs 22 and 29 will be found his last views on the life principle, which term he uses throughout, preferably to vital force as in former editions.

Paragraphs 52 to 56 have been wholly rewritten and long footnotes are added to Paragraphs 60-74. Again, Paragraph 148 is practically wholly new and concerns itself with the origin of disease, denying a *Materia peccans,* as the prime etiological factor.

Of greatest importance are Paragraphs 246-248 in regard to dosage in the treatment of chronic diseases. He there departs from the single dose and advises repetition of dosage but in different potencies. Paragraphs 269-272 are devoted to technical directions for the preparation of homœopathic medicines especially according to his latest views.

The vexed question of double remedies other than chemical compounds is fully and definitely settled in Paragraph 273 and all doubts as to the impropriety of such procedure removed.

Wholly new is the footnote to Paragraph 282 and of greatest importance. Here his treatment of the chronic diseases under psora, syphilis, and sycosis departs absolutely from that advised in former editions. He now advises to commence treatment with large doses of their specific remedies early and, if necessary, several times daily and gradually ascend to higher degrees of dynamization. In the treatment of figwarts the local application is considered necessary with the internal use of the remedy.

The book as now presented is Hahnemann's last word concerning the principles advanced by him in the first and subsequent editions, illuminated and enlarged by his vast experience in the latter part of his medical career in the treatment of both acute and chronic diseases. Historically, the book in its sixth edition is of the greatest interest and importance, completing as it does the marvelous array of Hahnemann's philosophic insight into the practice of medicine. Hahnemann's "Organon" is the high water mark of medical philosophy, the practical interpretation of which produces a veritable mountain of light and will guide the physician by means of the Law of Cure to a new world in therapeutics.

This edition is favored with an introduction by Dr. James Krauss, of Boston, the learned and scholarly student of Hahnemann, to whom I herewith desire to express my grateful appreciation for both the introduction and other valuable aid.

WILLIAM BOERICKE.

San Francisco, December, 1921.

INTRODUCTION

(To Doctor Boericke's translation of the sixth edition of
Hahnemann's "Organon.")

The excellence of the Dudgeon translation into English
of the fifth German edition of Hahnemann's "Organon"
is thoroughly maintained throughout this English translation of the sixth German edition by Doctor William
Boericke, to whom the medical profession is under a double debt for rescuing this last authentic work of Hahnemann from possible loss and for putting it into good,
clear, unparaphrased English. Twice, this manuscript of
Hahnemann was in danger of being lost, once during
the siege of Paris in the Franco-Prussian War of 1870-
71, and once in the military over-running of Westphalia
during the World War of 1914-18. Doctor Boericke was
the main instrument for procuring this last medical
manuscript of Hahnemann for the medical world.

Everything that Hahnemann ever wrote is of historic
medical interest, for notwithstanding all attempts of ignorant, prejudiced, time-serving so-called medical historians
to detract from Hahnemann his historic importance for
medicine, Hahnemann remains one of the four epochal
figures in the history of the practice of medicine. Hippocrates, the Observer, introduced the art of clinical observation as the necessary basis for pathologic diagnosis.
Galen, the Disseminator, spread with powerful authority
the teachings of Hippocrates over the medical world.
Paracelsus, the Assailer, introduced chemical as well as
physical analysis into the practice of medicine. Hahnemann, the Experimenter, discovered the symptomatic

source of both pathologic and therapeutic diagnosis and thereby made the practice of medicine scientific.

In the scientific practice of medicine, we examine every patient suffering from any of the topic, plastic, trophic and toxic diseases to which man is subject, in order to obtain all the signs and symptoms of his disease, all his disease effects for pathologic and therapeutic diagnosis and prognosis. We examine by observing the pathologic and comparing it with the physiologic for diagnostic interpretation, prognostic predication, and therapeutic application. We diagnose by classifying the pathologic condition with similar pathologic conditions. We diagnose the anatomic seat, the where, that is, the organs and the parts of the organs affected. We diagnose the physiologic process, the what, that is, the course of inflammations, exudations, degenerations, necroses, atrophies, hypertrophies, aplasias, hyperplasias. We diagnose the etiologic factor, the how, that is, developmental, traumatic, infectious antecedents of predisposition and excitation. We diagnose the therapeutic application, the end, that is, the remedial treatment for cure and palliation, and the prophylactic treatment for hygiene and sanitation.

The treatment of patients, subject to malformations, malpositions, malnutritions, injuries, foreign bodies, traumatic and infection inflammations, new formations, is effected with medical, surgical, hygienic means, or a combination of all these in a given patient. Surgery may remove or palliate effects of anatomic excesses, defects, perversions. Food, water, air, heat and cold, light and electricity, exercise and work, massage and suggestion, as well as glands to replace glands, vaccines to call out antibodies and sera to supply antibodies may remedy or palliate effects of physiologic excesses, deficiencies, perversions, may restore hygiene and establish sanitation. Medicine, in the form of medicinal substances, may remedy or palliate effects of etiologic excesses, defects, perversions, effects which are not remedied or remediable, palliated or palliable by surgery, hygienic or quasi-hygienic measures.

It is impossible to know all the antecedents causative of disease consequents. *Tolle causam* is easier said than done. How, then, shall we remove or palliate these effects by medical substances? Here, Hahnemann steps in to say, for the first time in all history: Remove the effects and you remove the disease, the cause of the effects. *Cessat effectus cessat causa.* Empiric medicine guesses, recommends, tries, hits and misses, misses and hits again. Scientific medicine does not guess. Scientific medicine, like any other scientific art, compares effects, sensations and motions with corresponding effects, corresponding sensations and motions. Only the mountebanks in medicine decry methods of comparison as unscientific. All that we can humanly do, and scientifically do do, is to observe and classify, to compare and infer. Hahnemann says, we must apply medicinal substances on the basis of knowledge of their actual effects. Since it is impossible to know all the antecedents causative of disease consequents, we must treat the disease effects which we do know by medicinal effects which we have ascertained and know. Disease effects are removed by the application of medicines having corresponding medicinal effects. If the disease effects are removed *in toto,* we have a cure. If the disease effects are removed in part, we have palliation. Scientific comparison of disease effects and medicinal effects for application leads to the diagnostic inferences of scientific medicine, makes scientific medicine possible.

In 1790, Hahnemann made his celebrated experiment with china. From that time to 1839, that is, in the course of about fifty years, he experimented with ninety-nine drugs and recorded his observations of their actions on the human body. This record, found in his "Fragmenta de Viribus Medicamentorum Positivis," "Materia Medica Pura" and "Chronic Diseases" is the largest, the most accurate and the most fertile of all investigations into medicinal action made by any single observer, before or since Hahnemann, throughout the annals of medical history.

Hahnemann was, in all essentials, a flawless experimenter. He took four drachms of china twice a day. He had paroxysms of chill and fever. In his practice as a physician he had seen similar paroxysms of chill and fever. He had cured them with china, the Peruvian bark. No longer might it be said that Peruvian bark cures paroxysms of chill and fever because it is a bitter or astringent drug. The true inference stood out boldly. Peruvian bark cures paroxysms of chills and fever because Peruvian bark produces paroxysms of chills and fever. The necessity for the methodical discovery of the medicinal properties of drugs was made apparent. He who says that Hahnemann should not have experimented on himself but on dogs, or cats, or rats, or mice, has not yet entered the school of scientific logic. Disease manifests itself not merely by objective signs of sensory impression, but also by subjective symptoms of motor expression. Can the human experimenter record the subjective feelings of dogs, and cats, and rats, and mice when the dogs, and cats, and rats, and mice cannot communicate to his understanding their subjective feelings? There are no two human beings entirely the same in health and disease. Are dogs, or cats, or mice, or rats more nearly like to human beings than human beings are like to one another?

The routine experimenter, or so-called experimenter, experiments as though experiments were ends in themselves. This is the reason for the sterility of most public and private experimental stations. The experimenter experiments, but does not know why he experiments. The moral justification may be that he experiments because he is paid to experiment; but where is the scientific justification? Hahnemann had scientific justification for his experiments. That is the reason why his experiments were not sterile.

Experimentation is for one of two purposes, observation for induction, or verification of inductions. Experimentation is analysis, deduction, analytic deduction. We deduce from objects of nature, man or drug, properties in contrast with other properties. We observe by contrast. Observation is comparison, weighing, judging of contrasts. We compare for correspondence. We classify by resemblance. Classification is synthesis, induction, synthetic induction. We classify, conceive for reflection, thought, judgment. We think for expression. We formulate our propositions for verification. We verify by experimentation, by analytic deduction, the formulated propositions of science, of scientific inductions.

Hahnemann experimented for observation. He perceived in himself the symptomatic effects of Peruvian bark as similar to the symptomatic effects of intermittent fever he had removed in others with Peruvian bark. Who can say that china, taken into the healthy human body, will not produce signs, objective symptoms and feelings, subjective symptoms similar to those of intermittent fever? Hahnemann had the contrast of health without the drug and disease with the drug within himself. He was not a sterile observer. Perception led at once to conception. Hahnemann conceived the symptomatic affinity of drugs for tissues, the symptomsimilarity of drugs and tissues as essential for the medical treatment of medically curable diseases. If ever there was a clear scientific induction from scientific observation, it was this induction of Hahnemann's symptomsimilarity of drugs and tissues, which he denominated homœopathy, and for the elucidation of which he wrote his "Organon of Medicine" in 1810, and re-wrote it consecutively in 1819, 1824, 1829, 1833, and finally annotated and emended the 1833 edition for this sixth, his last edition, in 1842.

Was he in error? Was he premature with his conception? Hahnemann was not one of those so-called scientists who collect and catalogue their perceptual facts with no more scientific imagination than is exercised by cataloguers of libraries and collectors of taxes. Science is verified or verifiable knowledge produced by conception of percepts, induction of deducts. For scientific imagination, conceptuation from perception, not many percepts are needed. Was Pythagoras in error because, perceiving mast and sails before perceiving the hull of a ship on the horizon, he conceived that the earth is round? Was his conception premature, untrue, because everybody except Aristotle for nearly two thousand years maintained that the earth is flat, because it took nearly two thousand years before Columbus began and Magellan finished the rounding of the earth?

Hahnemann himself saw to it that there was no error in his induction. He was his own Columbus, his own Magellan. Hahnemann treated, with his own hands, his own medically curable patients and taught other medical men to treat their own medically curable patients by the method of symptomsimilarity he had conceived. In 1797, he used veratrum album for colic, and nux vomica for asthma, and cured the multitudinous medically curable patients that came to him from his sojourn in Königslutter to his last abiding place in Paris by this method of symptomsimilarity, the central method of scientific medical therapeutics. His were truly scientific verifications. Those that doubt this really do not doubt. They know not what they doubt. The verifications of Hahnemann convince those who have intellectual integrity for scientific conviction, who will not sacrifice their intellectual integrity to the idols of the day, who will repeat Hahnemann's experimental verifications of his scientific observations and inductions as they should be repeated. Any other method than to take into the healthy body four drachms of china twice a day to prove or to disprove the symptomsimilarity of china and intermittent fever is not a scientific experiment for the observation of Hahnemann, that there is symptomsimilarity between china and intermittent fever. Any other method than to administer china to patients suffering from intermittent fever to prove or to disprove the method of symptomsimilarity in dosage smaller than that used for exciting the healthy body into disease action similar to that of intermittent fever is not a scientific experimental verification of the induction of Hahnemann, that symptomsimilarity is the curative method of medically curable diseases. Those that pursue other methods have not even the frogs' legs of Aristophanes to stand upon. Pasteur, perceiving that Jenner's milder cowpox prevented the appearance of the severer smallpox, conceived the prophylactic treatment of infectious diseases by milder vaccinations with the virus exciting a given infection. How did Pasteur prove his conception? He took a number of sheep; vaccinated some of the sheep with a milder prophylactic dose of anthrax virus; then injected into all the sheep anthrax virus in larger dosage sufficient to excite anthrax; all those sheep he had vaccinated previously with the milder prophylactic anthrax virus lived without anthrax; those not vaccinated prophylactically died with anthrax. Pasteur, like the elder and greater Hahnemann, was a scientific experimenter, not a would-be experimenter.

The era of scientific medical experimentation begins with Hahnemann and nobody else. Scientific to the core, Hahnemann experimented scientifically for scientific observation. Alert with intellectual power, he conceived his induction scientifically from scientific observation. Uncompromisingly scientific for experimental verification, he verified his induction scientifically for all time on his patients and made his method of symptomsimilarity for all time the central curative method of scientific medical therapeutics. For over a hundred years this method has been consciously and unconsciously followed by the medical profession. The results substantiate Hahnemann's contentions. There is no greater achievement than to have scientific truth, pass it on, have succeeding generations follow it and express it. Hahnemann's "Organon of Medicine" goes out to teach symptomsimilarity as the experimental basis of pathologic and therapeutic diagnosis, as the *echte Heilweg* of scientific medicine.

JAMES KRAUSS, M. D.

Boston, September 30, 1921.

AUTHOR'S PREFACE TO THE SIXTH EDITION.*

In order to give a general notion of the treatment of diseases pursued by the old school of medicine (allopathy) it may be observed that it presupposes the existence sometimes of excess of blood (*plethora—which is never present*), sometimes of morbid matters and acridities; hence it taps off the life's blood and exerts itself either to clear away the imaginary disease-matter or to conduct it elsewhere (by emetics, purgatives, sialogogues, diaphoretics, diuretics, drawing plasters, setons, issues, etc.), in the vain belief that the disease will thereby be weakened and materially eradicated; in place of which the patient's sufferings are thereby increased, and by such and other painful appliances the forces and nutritious juices indispensable to the curative process are abstracted from the organism. It assails the body with large doses of power-

---

* In Hahnemann's manuscript copy, he has a note in French which, translated is as follows:

Medicine as commonly practised (allopathy) knows no treatment except to draw from diseases the injurious materials which are assumed to be their cause. The blood of the patient is made to flow mercilessly by bleedings, leeches, cuppings, scarifications, to diminish an assumed plethora which never exists as in well women a few days before their menses, an accumulation of blood the loss of which is of no appreciable consequence, while the loss of blood with merely assumed plethora destroys life. Medicine as commonly practised seeks to evacuate the contents of the stomach and sweep the intestines clear of the materials assumed to originate diseases.

ful medicines, often repeated in rapid succession for a long time, whose long-enduring, not infrequently frightful effects it knows not, and which it, purposely it would almost seem, makes unrecognisable by the commingling of several such unknown substances in one prescription, and by their long-continued employment it develops in the body new and often ineradicable medicinal diseases. Whenever it can, it employs, in order to keep in favor with its patient,[1] remedies that immediately suppress and hide the morbid symptoms by opposition (*contraria contrariis*) for a short time (palliatives), but that leave the cause for these symptoms (the disease itself) strengthened and aggravated. It considers affections on the exterior of the body as purely local and existing there independently, and vainly supposes that it has cured them when it has driven them away by means of external remedies, so that the internal affection is thereby compelled to break out on a nobler and more important part. When it knows not what else to do for the disease which will not yield or which grows worse, the old school of medicine undertakes to change it into something else, it knows not what, by means of an *alterative*,—for example, by the life-undermining calomel, corrosive sublimate and other mercurial preparations in large doses.

It seems that the unhallowed principal business of the old school of medicine (allopathy) is to render in-

---

[1] For the same object the experienced allopath delights to invent a fixed name, by preference a Greek one, for the malady, in order to make the patient believe that he has long known this disease as an old acquaintance, and hence is the fitted person to cure it.

curable if not fatal the majority of diseases, those made chronic through ignorance by continually weakening and tormenting the already debilitated patient by the further addition of new destructive drug diseases. When this pernicious practice has become a habit and one is rendered insensible to the admonitions of conscience, this becomes a very easy business indeed.

And yet for all these mischievous operations the ordinary physician of the old school can assign his reasons, which, however, rest only on foregone conclusions of his books and teachers, and on the authority of this or that distinguished physician of the old school. Even the most opposite and the most senseless modes of treatment find there their defence, their authority—let their disastrous effects speak ever so loudly against them. It is only under the old physician who has been at last gradually convinced, after many years of misdeeds, of the mischievous nature of hi. so-called art, and who no longer treats even the severest diseases with anything stronger than plantain water mixed with strawberry syrup (*i. e.*, with nothing), that the smallest number are injured and die.

This non-healing art, which for many centuries has been firmly established in full possession of the power to dispose of the life and death of patients according to its own good will and pleasure, and in that period has shortened the lives of ten times as many human beings as the most destructive wars, and rendered many millions of patients more diseased and wretched than they were originally—this allopathy, I have, in the introduction to the former editions of this book, considered more in detail. Now I shall consider only its exact opposite, the true healing art, discovered by me and now somewhat more perfected. Examples are given to prove that striking cures performed in former times were always due to remedies basically homœopathic and found by the physician accidentally and contrary to the then prevailing methods of therapeutics.

As regards the latter (homœopathy) it is quite otherwise. It can easily convince every reflecting person that the diseases of man are not caused by any substance, any acridity, that is to say, any disease-matter, but that they are solely spirit-like (dynamic) derangements of the spirit-like power (the vital principle) that animates the human body. Homœopathy knows that a cure can only take place by the reaction of the vital force against the rightly chosen remedy that has been ingested, and that the cure will be certain and rapid in proportion to the strength with which the vital force still prevails in the patient. Hence homœopathy *avoids everything in the slightest degree enfeebling*,[2] and as much as possible every excitation of pain, for pain also diminishes the strength, and hence it employs for the cure ONLY those medicines whose power for altering and deranging (dynamically) the health it knows *accurately,* and from these it selects one whose pathogenetic power (its medicinal disease) is

---

[2] Homœopathy sheds not a drop of blood, administers no emetics, purgatives, laxatives or diaphoretics, drives off no external affection by external means, prescribes no hot or unknown mineral baths or medicated clysters, applies no Spanish flies or mustard plasters, no setons, no issues, excites no ptyalism, burns not with moxa or red-hot iron to the very bone, and so forth, but gives with its own hand its own preparations of simple uncompounded medicines, which it is accurately acquainted with, never subdues pain by opium, etc.

capable of removing the natural disease in question by similarity (*similia similibus*), and this it administers to the patient in simple form, but in rare and minute doses so small that, without occasioning pain or weakening, they just suffice to remove the natural malady whence this result: that without weakening, injuring or torturing him in the very least, the natural disease is extinguished, and the patient, even whilst he is getting better, gains in strength and thus is cured—an apparently easy but actually troublesome and difficult business, and one requiring much thought, but which restores the patient without suffering in a short time to perfect health,—and thus it is a salutary and blessed business.

Thus homœopathy is a perfectly simple system of medicine, remaining always fixed in its principles as in its practice, which, like the doctrine whereon it is based, if rightly apprehended will be found to be complete (and therefore serviceable). What is clearly pure in doctrine and practice should be self-evident, and all backward sliding to the pernicious routinism of the old school that is as much its antithesis as night is to day, should cease to vaunt itself with the honorable name of Homœopathy.

SAMUEL HAHNEMANN.

Köthen, March 28, 1833.
Confirmed Paris,   184—[a]

---

[a] Hahnemann did not put in his manuscript the exact date, leaving this probably until the book would go to the printer, but Dr. Haehl suggests February, 1842, as the date according to a manuscript copy made by Madame Hahnemann.

Wм. B.

CONTENTS.

INTRODUCTION.

Examples of accidental homœopathic cures.

Non-medical persons have also found the treatment on the principle of similarity of action to be the only efficacious mode.

Even some physicians of an earlier period suspected that this was the most excellent mode of treatment.

TEXT OF THE ORGANON.

§ 1, 2. The sole mission of the physician is to cure rapidly, gently, permanently.

> NOTE.—Not to construct theoretical systems, nor to attempt to explain phenomena.

3, 4. He must investigate what is to be cured in disease and know what is curative in the various medicines, in order to be able to adapt the latter to the former, and must also understand how to preserve the health of human beings.

5. Attention to exciting and fundamental causes and other circumstances, as helps to cure.

6. For the physician, the disease consists only of the totality of its symptoms.

> NOTE.—The old school's futile attempts to discover the essential nature of disease (*prima causa*).

7. Whilst paying attention to those circumstances (§ 5) the physician needs only to remove the totality of the symptoms in order to cure the disease.

> NOTE 1.—The cause that manifestly produces and maintains the disease should be removed.

> NOTE 2.—The symptomatic palliative mode of treatment directed towards a single symptom is to be rejected.

INTRODUCTION.

Review of the therapeutics, allopathy and palliative treatment that have hitherto been practiced in the old school of medicine.

As long as men have existed they have been liable, individually or collectively, to diseases from physical or moral causes. In a rude state of nature but few remedial agents were required, as the simple mode of living admitted of but few diseases; with the civilization of mankind in the state, on the contrary, the occasions of diseases and the necessity for medical aid increased in equal proportion. But ever since that time (soon after Hippocrates, therefore, for 2500 years) men have occupied themselves with the treatment of the ever increasing multiplicity of diseases, who, led astray by their vanity, sought by reasoning and guessing to excogitate the mode of furnishing this aid. Innumerable and dissimilar ideas respecting the nature of diseases and their remedies sprang from so many dissimilar brains, and the theoretical views these gave rise to the so-called *systems,* each of which was at variance with the rest and self-contradictory. Each of these subtile expositions at first threw the readers into stupefied amazement at the incomprehensible wisdom contained in it, and attracted to the system-monger a number of followers, who re-echoed his unnatural sophistry, to none of whom, however, was it of the slightest use in enabling them to cure better, until a new system, often diametrically opposed to the first, thrust that aside, and in its turn gained a short-lived renown. None of them, however, was in consonance with nature and ex-

(30)

perience; they were mere theoretical webs, woven by cunning intellects out of pretended consequences, which could not be made use of in practice, in the treatment at the sick-bed, on account of their excessive subtilty and repugnance to nature, and only served for empty disputations.

Simultaneously, but quite independent of all these theories, there sprung up a mode of treatment with mixtures of unknown medicinal substances for forms of disease arbitrarily set up, and directed towards some material object completely at variance with nature and experience, hence, as may be supposed, with a bad result—such is old medicine, *allopathy* as it is termed.

Without disparaging the services which many physicians have rendered to the sciences auxiliary to medicine, to natural philosophy and chemistry, to natural history in its various branches, and to that of man in particular, to anthropology, physiology and anatomy, etc., I shall occupy myself here with the practical part of medicine only, with the healing art itself, in order to show how it is that diseases have hitherto been so imperfectly treated. Far beneath my notice is that mechanical routine of treating precious human life according to the prescription manuals, the continual publication of which shows, alas! how frequently they are still used. I pass it by unnoticed, as a despicable practice of the lowest class of ordinary practitioners. I speak merely of the medical art as hitherto practiced, which, pluming itself on its antiquity, imagines itself to possess a scientific character.

The partisans of the old school of medicine flattered themselves that they could justly claim for it alone the title of *"rational medicine,"* because they alone sought for and strove to remove the *cause of disease, and followed the method employed by nature in diseases.*

Tolle causam! they cried incessantly. But they went no further than this empty exclamation. *They only fancied* that they could discover the cause of disease; they did not discover it, however, as it is not perceptible and not discoverable. For as far the greatest number of diseases are of dynamic (spiritual) origin and dynamic (spiritual) nature, their cause is therefore not perceptible to the senses; so they exerted themselves to imagine one, and from a survey of the parts of the normal, inanimate human body (anatomy), compared with the visible changes of the same internal parts in persons who had died of diseases (pathological anatomy), as also from what they could deduce from a comparison of the phenomena and functions in healthy life (physiology) with their endless alterations in the innumerable morbid states (pathology, semeiotics), to draw conclusions relative to the invisible process whereby the changes which take place in the *inward* being of man in diseases are affected—a dim picture of the imagination, which theoretical medicine regarded as its *prima causa morbi;*[1] and thus it was at

---

[1] It would have been much more consonant with sound human reason and with the nature of things, had they, in order to be able to cure a disease, regarded the originating cause as the *causa morbi,* and endeavored to discover that, and thus been enabled successfully to employ the mode of treatment which had shown itself useful in maladies having the same exciting cause, in those also of a similar origin, as, for example, the same mercury is efficacious in an ulcer of the glans after impure coitus, as in all previous venereal chancres—if, I say, they had discov-

one and the same time *the proximate cause of the disease,* and the internal essence of the disease, *the disease itself* —although, as sound human reason teaches us, the cause of a thing or of an event, can never be at the same time the thing or the event itself. How could they then, without deceiving themselves, consider this imperceptible internal essence as the object to be treated, and prescribe for it medicines whose curative powers were likewise generally unknown to them, and even give several such unknown medicines mixed together in what are termed prescriptions?

But this sublime problem, the discovery, namely, *a priori,* of an internal invisible cause of disease, resolved itself, at least with the more astute physicians of the old

---

ered the exciting cause of all other (non-venereal) chronic diseases to be an infection at one period or another with the itch miasm (*psora*), and had found for all these a common method of treatment, regard being had for the peculiarities of each individual case, whereby all and each of these chronic diseases might have been cured, then might they with justice have boasted that in the treatment of chronic diseases they had in view the *only available* and useful *causa morborum chronicorum* (*non venereorum*), and with this as a basis they might have treated such diseases with the best results. But during these many centuries they were unable to cure the millions of chronic diseases, because they knew not their origin in the psoric miasm (which was first discovered and afterwards provided with a suitable plan of treatment by homœopathy), and yet they vaunted that they alone kept in view the *prima causa* of these diseases in their treatment, and that they alone treated rationally, although they had not the slightest conception of the only useful knowledge of their psoric origin and consequently they bungled the treatment of all chronic diseases!

school, into a search, under the guidance of the symptoms it is true, for what might be supposed to be the probable general *character* of the case of disease before them;[2] whether it was spasm, or debility, or paralysis, or fever, or inflammation, or induration, or obstruction of this or that part, or excess of blood (plethora), deficiency or excess of oxygen, carbon, hydrogen or nitrogen in the juices, exaltation or depression of the functions of the arterial, venous or capillary system, change in the relative proportion of the factors of sensibility, irritability or reproduction?—conjectures that have been dignified by the followers of the old school with the title of causal indication, and considered to be the only possible rationality in medicine; but which were assumptions, too fallacious and hypothetical to prove of any practical utility—incapable, even had they been well grounded, of indicating the most appropriate remedy for a case of disease; flattering indeed, to the vanity of the learned theorist, but usually leading astray when used as guides to practice, and wherein there was evidenced more of ostentation than of an earnest search for the curative indication.

And how often has it happened that, for example, spasm or paralysis seemed to be in one part of the organism, while in another part inflammation was apparently present!

---

[2] Every physician who treats disease according to such general character however he may affect to claim the name of homœopathist, is and ever will remain in fact a generalising allopath, for without the most minute individualisation, homœopathy is not conceivable.

Or, on the other hand, whence are the certain remedies for each of these pretended general characters to be derived? Those that would certainly be of benefit could be none other than the *specific* medicines, that is, those whose action is homogeneous [3] to the morbid irritation; whose employment, however, is denounced and forbidden [4] by the old school as highly injurious, because observation has shown that in consequence of the receptivity for homogeneous irritation being so highly increased in diseases, such medicines in the usual large doses are dangerous to life. The old school never dreamt of smaller, and of extremely small doses. Accordingly no attempt was made to cure, in the direct (the most natural) way, by means of homogeneous, specific medicines; nor could it be done, as the effects of most of medicines were, and continued to remain, unknown, and even had they been known it would have been impossible to hit on the right medicine with such generalizing views as were entertained.

However, perceiving that it was more consistent with reason to seek for another path, a straight one if pos-

---

[3] Homœopathic.

[4] "Where experience showed the curative power of homœopathically acting remedies, whose mode of action could not be explained, the difficulty was avoided by calling them *specific*, and further investigation was stifled by this actually unmeaning word. The homogeneous excitant remedies, the specific (homœopathic), medicines, however, had long previously been prohibited as of very injurious influence."—Rau, *On the Value of the Homœopathic Method of Treatment*, Heidelberg, 1824, pp. 101, 102.

sible, rather than to take circuitous courses, the old school of medicine believed it might cure diseases in a direct manner by the *removal of the* (imaginary) *material cause of disease*—for to physicians of the ordinary school, while investigating and forming a judgment upon a disease, and not less while seeking for the curative indication, it was next to impossible to divest themselves of these materialistic ideas, and to regard the nature of the spiritual-corporeal organism as such a highly potentialized entity, that its sensational and functional vital changes, which are called diseases, must be produced and effected chiefly, if not solely, by dynamic (spiritual) influences, and could not be effected in any other way.

The old school regarded all those matters which **were** altered by the disease, those abnormal matters that occurred in congestions, as well as those that were excreted, as disease-producers, or at least on account of their supposed reacting power, as disease maintainers, and this latter notion prevails to this day.

Hence they dreamed of effecting causal cures by endeavoring to remove these imaginary and presumed material causes of the disease. Hence their assiduous evacuation of the bile by vomiting in bilious fevers; their emetics in cases of so-called stomach derangements;[5] their

---

[5] In a case of sudden derangement of the stomach, with constant disgusting eructations with the taste of the vitiated food, generally accompanied by depression of spirits, cold hands and feet, etc., the ordinary physician has hitherto been in the habit of attacking only the degenerated contents of the stomach; a powerful emetic should clean it out completely. This object was generally attained by tartar emetic, with or without ipecacu-

diligent purging away of the mucus, the lumbrici and
the ascarides in children who are pale-faced and who

---

anha. Does the patient, however, immediately after this become
well, brisk and cheerful? Oh, no! Such a derangement of the
stomach is usually of *dynamic origin,* caused by mental disturbance (grief, fright, vexation), a chill, over-exertion of the
mind or body immediately after eating, often after even a
moderate meal. Those two remedies are not suitable for removing this dynamic derangement, and just as little is the revolutionary vomiting they produce. Moreover, tartar emetic and
ipecacuanha, from their other peculiar pathogenetic powers, prove
of further injury to the patient's health, and derange the biliary
secretion; so that if the patient be not very robust, he must
feel ill for *several* days from the effects of this pretended causal
treatment, notwithstanding all this violent expulsion of the whole
contents of the stomach. If the patient, however, in place of
taking such violent and always (a) hurtful evacuant drugs, smell
only a single time at a globule the size of a mustard seed, moistened with highly diluted *pulsatilla* juice, whereby the derangement
of his health in general and of his stomach in particular will certainly be removed, in two hours he is quite well; and if the eructa-
tion recur once more, it consists of tasteless and inodorous air;
the contents of the stomach cease to be vitiated, and at the next
meal he has regained his full usual appetite; he is quite well and
lively. This is true causal medication; the former is only an
imaginary one and has an injurious effect on the patient.

Even a stomach overloaded with indigestible food *never* requires a medicinal emetic. In such a case nature is competent to
rid herself of the excess in the best way through the œsophagus,
by means of nausea, sickness and spontaneous vomiting, assisted,
it may be, by mechanical irritation of the palate and fauces, and
by this means the accessory medicinal effects of the emetic drugs
are avoided; a small quantity of coffee expedites the passage
downwards of what remains in the stomach.

But if, after excessive overloading of the stomach, the irritability of the stomach is not sufficient to promote spontaneous vomit-

suffer from ravenous appetite, bellyache, and enlarged abdomen;[6] their venesections in cases of hæmorrhage;[7]

---

ing, or is lost altogether, so that the tendency thereto is extinguished, while there are at the same time great pains in the epigastrium, in such a paralyzed state of the stomach, an emetic medicine would only have the effect of producing a dangerous or fatal inflammation of the intestines; where a small quantity of strong infusion of coffee, frequently administered, would dynamically exalt the sunken irritability of the stomach, and put it in a condition to expel its contents, be they ever so great, either upwards or downwards. So here also the pretended causal treatment is out of place.

Even the acrid gastric acid, to eructations of which patients with chronic diseases are not infrequently subject, may be today violently evacuated by means of an emetic, with great suffering, and yet all in vain, for tomorrow or some days later it is replaced by similar acrid gastric acid, and then usually in larger quantities; whereas it goes away by itself when its dynamic cause is removed by a very small dose of a high dilution of *sulphuric acid,* or still better, if it is of frequent recurrence, by the employment of minutest doses of antipsoric remedies corresponding in similarity to the rest of the symptoms also. And of a similar character are many of the pretended causal cures of the old-school physicians, whose main effort it is, by means of tedious operations, troublesome to themselves and injurious to their patients, to clear away the material product of the dynamic derangement; whereas if they perceived the dynamic source of the affection, and annihilated it and its products homœopathically, they would thereby effect a rational *cure.*

[6] Conditions dependent solely on a psoric taint, and easily curable by mild (dynamic) antipsoric remedies without emetics or purgatives.

[7] Notwithstanding that almost all morbid hæmorrhages depend on a dynamic derangement of the vital force (state of health), yet the old-school physicians consider their cause to be excess of blood, and cannot refrain from bleeding in order to draw off the

and more especially all their varieties of blood-lettings,[8] their main remedy in inflammations, which they now, following the example of a well-known bloodthirsty Parisian physician (as a flock of sheep follow the bell-wether even into the butcher's slaughter-house), imagine to encounter in almost every morbidly affected part of

---

supposed superabundance of this vital fluid; the palpable evil consequences of which procedure, however, such as prostration of the strength, and the tendency, or actual transition, to the typhoid state they ascribe to the malignancy of the disease, *which they are then often unable to overcome*—in fine, they imagine, even when the patient does not recover, that their treatment has been in conformity with their axiom, *causam tolle,* and that, according to their mode of speaking, they have done everything in their power for the patient, let the result be what it may.

[8] Although there probably never was a drop of blood too much in the living human body, yet the old-school practitioners consider an imaginary excess of blood as the main material cause of all hæmorrhages and inflammations, which they must remove and drain off by venesections, cupping and leeches. This they hold to be a rational mode of treatment, causal medication. In general inflammatory fevers, in acute pleurisy, they even regard the coagulable lymph in the blood—the buffy coat, as it is termed—as the *materia peccans,* which they endeavor to get rid of, if possible, by repeated venesections, notwithstanding that this coat often becomes more consistent and thicker at every repetition of the bloodletting. They thus often bleed the patient nearly to death, when the inflammatory fever will not subside, in order to remove this buffy coat or the imaginary plethora, without suspecting that the inflammatory blood is only the product of the acute fever, of the morbid, immaterial (dynamic) inflammatory irritation, and that the latter is the sole cause of the great disturbance in the vascular system, and may be removed by the smallest dose of a homogeneous (homœopathic) medicine, as,

the body, and feel themselves, bound to remove by the application of often a fatal number of leeches. They believe that by so doing they obey the true casual indications, and treat disease in a rational manner. The adherents of the old school, moreover, believe that by putting a ligature on polypi, by cutting out, or artificially exciting suppuration by means of local irritants in indolent gland-

---

for instance, by a small globule of the decillion-fold dilution of *aconite* juice, with abstinence from vegetable acids, so that *the most violent pleuritic fever*, with all its alarming concomitants, is changed into health *and cured, without the least abstraction of blood and without any antiphlogistic remedy, in a few*—at the most *in twenty-four*—hours (a small quantity of blood drawn from a vein by the way of experiment then shows no traces of buffy coat); whereas another patient similarly affected, and treated on the rational principles of the old school, if, after repeated bleedings, with great difficulty and unspeakable sufferings he escape for the nonce with life, he often has still many months to drag through before he can support his emaciated body on his legs, if in the mean time (as often happens from such maltreatment) he be not carried off by typhoid fever, leucophlegmasia or pulmonary phthisis.

Anyone who has felt the tranquil pulse of a man an hour before the occurrence of the rigor that always precedes an attack of acute pleurisy, will not be able to restrain his amazement if told two hours later, after the hot stage has commenced, that the enormous plethora present urgently requires repeated venesections, and will naturally inquire by what magic power could the pounds of blood that must now be drawn off have been conjured into the blood-vessels of this man within these two hours, which but two hours previously he had felt beating in such a tranquil manner. Not a single drachm more of blood can now be circulating in those vessels than existed when he was in good health, not yet two hours ago!

ular swellings, by enucleating encysted tumors (steatoma and meliceria) by their operations for aneurysm and lacrymal and anal fistula, by removing with the knife scirrhous tumors of the breast, by amputating a limb

---

Accordingly the allopathic physician with his venesections draws from the patient laboring under acute fever no oppressive superabundance of blood, as that cannot possibly be present; he only robs him of what is indispensable to life and recovery, the normal quantity of blood and consequently of strength —a great loss which no physician's power can replace!—and yet he vainly imagines that he has conducted the treatment in conformity to his (misunderstood) axiom, *causam tolle;* whereas it is impossible that the *causa morbi* in this case can be an excess of blood, which is not present; but the sole true *causa morbi* was a morbid, dynamical, inflammatory irritation of the circulatory system, as is proved by the rapid and permanent cure of this *and every similar case* of general inflammatory fever by one or two inconceivably minute doses of *aconite* juice, which removes such an irritation homœopathically.

The old school errs equally in the treatment of local inflammations with its topical bloodlettings, more especially with the quantities of leeches which are now applied according to the maniacal principles of Broussais. The palliative amelioration that at first ensues from the treatment is far from being crowned by a rapid and perfect cure; on the contrary, the weak and ailing state of the parts thus treated (frequently also of the whole body), which always remains, sufficiently shows the error that is committed in attributing the local inflammation to a local plethora, and how sad are the consequences of such abstractions of blood; whereas this purely dynamic, apparently local, inflammatory irritation, can be rapidly and permanently removed by an equally small dose of *aconite,* or, according to circumstances, of *belladonna,* and the whole disease annihilated and cured, without such unjustifiable shedding of blood.

affected with necrosis, etc., they cure the patient radically, and that their treatment is directed against the cause
of the disease; and they also think, when they employ
their *repellent* remedies, dry up old running ulcers in the
legs with astringent applications of oxide of lead, cop-
per or zinc (aided always by the simultaneous administration of purgatives, which merely debilitate, but have no
effect on the fundamental dyscrasia), cauterize chancres,
destroy condylomata locally, drive off itch from the skin
with ointments of sulphur, oxide of lead, mercury or
zinc, suppress ophthalmiæ with solutions of lead or
zinc, and drive away tearing pains from the limbs by
means of opodeldoc, hartshorn liniment or fumigations
with cinnabar or amber; in every case they think they
have removed the affection, conquered the disease, and
pursued a rational treatment directed towards the cause.
But *what is the result?* The metastatic affections that
sooner or later, but inevitably appear, caused by this
mode of treatment (but which they pretend are entirely
new diseases), *which are always worse than the original
malady,* sufficiently prove their error, and might and
should open their eyes to the deeper-seated, immaterial
nature of the disease, and its dynamic (spirit-like) origin,
which can only be removed by dynamic means.

A favorite idea of the ordinary school of medicine,
until recent (would that I could not say the most recent)
times, was that of morbific matters (and acridities) in
diseases, excessively subtile though they might be thought
to be, which must be expelled from the blood-vessels and
lymphathics, through the exhalents, skin, urinary apparatus
or salivary glands, through the tracheal and bronchial
glands in the form of expectoration, from the stomach

and bowels by vomiting and purging, in order that the body might be freed from the material cause that produced the disease, and a radical causal treatment be thus carried out.

By cutting holes in the diseased body, which were converted into chronic ulcers kept up for years by the introduction of foreign substances (issues, setons), they sought to draw off the *materia peccans* from the (always only dynamically) diseased body, just as one lets a dirty fluid run out of a barrel through the tap-hole. By means also of perpetual fly-blisters and the application of mezereum, they thought to draw away the bad humors and to cleanse the diseased body from all morbific matters—but they only weakened it, so as generally to render it incurable, by all these senseless unnatural processes.

I admit that it was more convenient for the weakness of humanity to assume that, in the diseases they were called on to cure, there existed some morbific material of which the mind might form a conception (more particularly as the patients readily lent themselves to such a notion), because in that case the practitioner had nothing further to care about than to procure a good supply of remedies for purifying the blood and humors, exciting diuresis and diaphoresis, promoting expectoration, and scouring out the stomach and bowels. Hence, in all the works on *Materia Medica,* from Dioscorides down to the latest books on this subject, there is almost nothing said about the special peculiar action of individual medicines; but, besides on account of their supposed utility in various nosological names of diseases, it is merely stated whether they are diuretic, diaphoretic, expectorant or emmenagogue, and more particularly whether they produce evacuation of the stomach and bowels upwards or downwards; because all the aspirations and efforts of the practitioner have ever been chiefly directed to cause the expulsion of a material morbific matter, and of sundry (fictitious) acridities, which it was imagined were the cause of diseases.

These were, however, all idle dreams, unfounded assumptions and hypotheses, cunningly devised for the convenience of therapeutics, as it was expected the easiest way of performing a cure would be to remove the material morbific matters (*si modo essent!*).

But the essential nature of diseases and their cure will not adapt themselves to such fantasies, nor to the convenience of medical men; to humor such stupid baseless hypotheses diseases will not cease to be (spiritual) *dynamic derangements of our spirit-like vital principle in sensations and functions, that is to say, immaterial derangements of our state of health.*

The causes of our maladies cannot be material, since the least foreign material substance,[9] however mild it may appear to us, if introduced into our blood-vessels, is promptly ejected by the vital force, as though it were a poison; or when this does not happen, death ensues. If

---

[9] Life was endangered by injecting a little pure water into a vein. (*Vide* Mullen, quoted by Birch in the *History of the Royal Society.*)

Atmospheric air injected into the blood-vessels caused death. (*Vide* J. M. Voigt, *Magazin für den neuesten Zustand der Naturkunde,* i, iii, p. 25.)

Even the mildest fluids introduced into the veins endangered life. (*Vide* Autenreith, *Physiologie,* ii, § 784.)

even the minutest splinter penetrates a sensitive part of our organism, the vital principle everywhere present in our body never rests until it is removed by pain, fever, suppuration or gangrene. And can it be supposed that in a case of cutaneous disease of twenty years' standing, for instance, this indefatigably active vital principle will quietly endure the presence of such an injurious foreign, material exanthematous substance, such as a herpetic, a scrofulous, a gouty acridity, etc., in the fluids of the body? Did any nosologist ever see with corporeal eyes such a morbific matter, to warrant him in speaking so confidently about it, and in founding a system of medical treatment upon it? Has any one ever succeeded in displaying to view the matter of gout or the poison of scrofula?

Even when the application of a material substance to the skin, or to a wound, has propagated diseases by infection, who can prove (what is so often maintained in works on pathology) that some material portion of this substance has penetrated into our fluids or been absorbed?[10] The most careful and prompt washing of the genitals does not protect the system from infection with the venereal chancrous disease. The slightest breath of air emanating from the body of a person affected with smallpox will suffice to produce this horrible disease in a healthy child.

---

[10] A girl in Glasgow, eight years of age, having been bit by a mad dog, *the surgeon immediately cut the piece clean out,* and yet thirty-six days afterwards she was seized with hydrophobia, which killed her in two days. (*Med. Comment. of Edinb.,* Dec. 2, vol. ii, 1793.)

What ponderable quantity of material substance could have been absorbed into the fluids, in order to develop, in the first of these instances, a tedious dyscrasia (syphilis), which when uncured is only extinguished with the remotest period of life, with death; in the last, a disease (smallpox) accompanied by almost general suppuration,[11] and often rapidly fatal? In these and all similar cases is it possible to entertain the idea of a material morbific matter being introduced into the blood? A letter written

---

[11] In order to account for the large quantity of putrid excrementitious matter and fœtid discharge often met with in diseases, and to be able to represent them as the material substance that excites and keeps up disease—although, when infection occurs, nothing perceptible in the shape of miasm, nothing material, could have penetrated into the body—recourse was had to the hypothesis, that the matter of infection, be it ever so minute, acts in the body like a ferment, bringing the fluids into a like state of corruption, and thus changing them into a similar morbific ferment which constantly increases with the disease and keeps it up. But by what all-potent and all-wise purifying draughts will you purge and cleanse the human fluids from this ever reproductive ferment, from this mass of imaginary morbific matter, and that so perfectly, that there shall not remain a particle of such morbific ferment, which, according to this hypothesis, must ever again, as at first, transform and corrupt the fluids to new morbific matter? Were that so it would evidently be impossible to cure these diseases in your way!—See how all hypotheses, be they ever so ingeniously framed, lead to the most palpable absurdities when they are not founded on truth!—The most deeply rooted syphilis may be cured, after the removal of the psora with which it is often complicated, by one or two small doses of the decillionfold diluted and potentised solution of *mercury,* whereby the general syphilitic taint of the fluids is forever (dynamically) annihilated and removed.

in the sick-room at a great distance has often communicated the same contagious disease to the person who read it. In this instance, can the notion of a material morbific matter having penetrated into the fluids be admitted? But what need is there of all such proofs? How often has it happened that an irritating word has brought on a dangerous bilious fever; a superstitious prediction of death has caused the fatal catastrophe at the very time announced; the abrupt communication of sad or excessively joyful news has occasioned sudden death? In these cases, where is the material morbific principle that entered in substance into the body, there to produce and keep up the disease, and without the material expulsion and ejection of which a radical cure were impossible?

The champions of this clumsy doctrine of morbific matters ought to be ashamed that they have so inconsiderately overlooked and failed to appreciate the spiritual nature of life, and the spiritual dynamic power of the exciting causes of diseases, and that they have thereby degraded themselves into mere scavenger-doctors, who, in their efforts to expel from the diseased body morbific matters that never existed, in place of curing, destroy life.

Are, then, the foul, often disgusting excretions which occur in diseases the actual matter that produces and keeps them up? [12] Are they not rather *always excretory products of the disease itself, that is, of the life which is only dynamically deranged and disordered?*

---

[12] Were this the case, the most inveterate coryza should be certainly and rapidly cured by merely blowing and wiping the nose carefully.

With such false and materialistic views concerning the origin and essential nature of diseases, it was certainly not to be wondered at that in all ages the main endeavor of the most obscure, as well as of the most distinguished practitioners, and even of the inventors of the sublimest medical systems, was always only to separate and expel an imaginary morbific matter, and the indication most frequently laid down was to break up and put in motion this morbific matter, to effect its expulsion by salivation, expectoration, diaphoresis and diuresis, to purify the blood from (acridities and impurities) morbific matters, *which never existed,* by means of the intelligence of sundry obedient decoctions of root and plants; to draw off mechanically the imaginary matter of disease by setons, by issues, by portions of the skin kept open and discharging by means of perpetual blisters or mezereum bark, but chiefly to expel and purge away the *materia peccans,* or the injurious matters as they were termed, through the intestines, by means of laxative and purgative medicines, which, in order to give them a more profound meaning and a more prepossessing appearance, were fondly denominated *dissolvents* and *mild aperients*—all so many arrangements for the expulsion of inimical morbific matters, which never could be, and never were instrumental in the production and maintenance of the diseases of the human organism, animated as it is by a spiritual principle—of diseases which never were anything else than spiritual dynamic derangements of the life altered in its sensations and functions.

Let it be granted now, what cannot be doubted, that no diseases—if they do not result from the introduction of perfectly indigestible or otherwise injurious substances into the stomach, or into other orifices or cavities of the body, or from foreign bodies penetrating the skin, etc.— that no disease, in a word, is caused by any material substance, but that every one is only and always a peculiar, virtual, dynamic derangement of the health; how injudicious, in that case, must not a method of treatment directed towards the expulsion [13] of that imaginary material

---

[13] There is a semblance of necessity in the expulsion by purgatives of worms, in so-called vermicular diseases. But even this semblance is false. A few lumbrici may be found in some children; in many there exist ascarides. But the presence of these is always dependent on a general taint of the constitution (the psoric), joined to an unhealthy mode of living. Let the latter be improved, and the former cured homœopathically, which is most easily effected at this age, and none of the worms remain, and children cured in this manner are never troubled with them more; whereas after mere purgatives, even when combined with cina seeds, they soon reappear in quantities.

"But the tapeworm," methinks I hear some one exclaim, "every effort should be made to expel that monster, which was created for the torment of mankind."

Yes, *sometimes* it is expelled; but at the cost of what after-sufferings, and with what danger to life! I should not like to have on my conscience the deaths of so many hundreds of human beings as have fallen sacrifices to the horribly violent purgatives, directed against the tapeworm, or the many years of indisposition of those who have escaped being purged to death. And how often does it happen that after all this health-and-life-destroying purgative treatment, frequently continued for several years, the animal is not expelled, or if so, that it is again produced!

What if there is not the slightest necessity for all these violent, cruel, and dangerous efforts to expel and kill the worm? The various species of tapeworm are only found along with the psoric taint, and always disappear when that is cured. But

substance appear to every rational man, since no good, but only monstrous harm, can result from its employment in the principal diseases of mankind, namely, those of a chronic character!

In short, the degenerated substances and impurities that appear in diseases are, undeniably, nothing more

---

even before the cure is accomplished, they live—the patient enjoying tolerable health the while—not exactly in the intestines, but in the residue of the food, the excrement of the bowels, as in their proper element, quite quietly, and without causing the least disturbance, and find in the excrement what suffices for their nourishment; they then do not touch the walls of the intestine, and are perfectly harmless. But if the patient happens to be affected with an acute disease of any kind, then the contents of the bowels become intolerable to the animal; it twists about, comes in contact with, and irritates the sensitive walls of the intestines, causing a peculiar kind of spasmodic colic, which increases materially the sufferings of the patient. (So also the fœtus in the womb becomes restless, turns about and kicks, only when the mother is ill; but when she is well, it swims quiet in its proper fluid without causing her any suffering.)

It is worthy of remark, that the morbid symptoms of patients suffering from tapeworm are generally of such a kind, that they are rapidly relieved (homœopathically) by the smallest dose of tincture of *male-fern root;* so that the ill-health of the patient, which causes this parasitic animal to be restless, is thereby for the time removed; the tapeworm then feels at ease, and lives on quietly in the excrement of the bowels, without particularly distressing the patient or his intestines, until the antipsoric treatment is so far advanced that the worm, after the eradication of the psora, finds the contents of the bowels no longer suitable for its support, and therefore spontaneously disappears, for ever from the now cured patient, without the least purgative medicine.

than products of the disease of the abnormally deranged organism, which are expelled by the latter, often violently enough—often much too violently—without requiring the aid of the evacuating art, and fresh products are always developed as long as it labors under that disease. These matters the true physician regards as actual symptoms of the disease, and they aid him to discover the nature of the disease, and to form an accurate portrait of it, so as to enable him to cure it with a similar medicinal morbific agent.

But the more modern adherents of the old school do not wish it to be supposed, that in their treatment they aim at the expulsion of material morbific substances. They allege that their multifarious evacuant processes are a mode of treatment by *derivation,* wherein they follow the example of nature which, in her efforts to assist the diseased organism, resolves fever by perspiration and diuresis pleurisy by epistaxis, sweat and mucous expectoration—other diseases by vomiting, diarrhœa and bleeding from the anus, articular pains by suppurating ulcers on the legs, cynanche tonsillaris by salivation, etc., or removes them by metastases and abscesses which she develops in parts at a distance from the seat of the disease.

Hence they thought the best thing to do was to *imitate* nature, by also going to work in the treatment of most diseases in a circuitous manner like the diseased vital force when left to itself and thus in an indirect manner,[14]

---

[14] In place of extinguishing the disease rapidly, without exhaustion of the strength and without going about the bush, with homogeneous, dynamic medicinal agents acting directly on the diseased points of the organism, as homœopathy does.

by means of stronger heterogeneous irritants applied to organs remote from the seat of disease, and totally dissimilar to the affected tissues, they produce evacuations, and generally kept them up, in order to *draw,* as it were, the disease thither.

This derivation, as it is called, was and continues to be one of the principal modes of treatment of the old school of medicine.

In this imitation of the self-aiding operation of nature, as some call it, they endeavored to excite, by force, new symptoms in the tissues that are least diseased and best able to bear the medicinal disease, which should draw away [15] the primary disease under the semblance of crises and under the form of excretions, in order to admit of a gradual lysis by the curative powers of nature.[16]

---

[15] Just as if anything immaterial could be drawn away! So that here too was the notion of a substance and a morbific matter, excessively subtile though it might be supposed to be!

[16] It is only the slighter and acute diseases that tend, when the natural period of their course has expired, to terminate quietly in resolution, as it is called, with or without the employment of not very aggressive allopathic remedies; the vital force, having regained its powers, then gradually substitutes the normal condition for the derangement of the health that has now ceased to exist. But in severe acute and in chronic diseases which constitute by far the greater portion of all human ailments, crude nature and the old school are equally powerless; in these, neither the vital force, with its self-aiding faculty, nor allopathy in imitation of it, can affect a lysis, but at the most a mere temporary truce, during which the enemy fortifies himself, in order, sooner or later, to recommence the attack with still greater violence

This they accomplished by means of diaphoretic and diuretic remedies, blood-lettings, setons and issues, but chiefly by irritant drugs to cause evacuation of the alimentary canal, sometimes upwards by means of emetics, sometimes (and this was the favorite plan) downwards by means of purgatives, which were termed aperient and dissolvent [17] remedies.

To assist this derivative method they employed the allied treatment by *counter-irritants;* woolen garments to the bare skin, foot-baths, nauseants, inflicting on the stomach and bowels the pangs of hunger (the hunger-treatment), substances to cause pain, inflammation, and suppuration in near or distant parts as the application of horseradish, mustard plasters, cantharides, blisters, mezereum setons, issues, tartar-emetic ointment, moxa, actual cautery, acupuncture, etc.; here also following the example of crude unassisted nature, which endeavors to free herself from the dynamic disease (in the case of a chronic disease, unavailingly) by exciting pain in distant parts of the body, by metastases and abscesses, by eruptions and suppurating ulcers.

It was evidently no rational principle, but merely *imitation,* with the view of making practice easy that seduced the old school into those unhelpful and injurious indirect modes of treatment, the derivative as well as the counter-irritant; that led them to this inefficacious, debilitating and hurtful practice of apparently ameliorating diseases

---

[17] An expression which likewise betrays that they imagined and presupposed a morbific substance, which had to be dissolved and expelled.

for a short time, or removing them in such a manner that another and a worse disease was roused up to occupy the place of the first. Such a destructive plan cannot certainly be termed curing.

They merely followed the example of crude instinctive nature in her efforts, which are barely [18] successful even

---

[18] In the ordinary school of medicine, the efforts made by nature for the relief of the organism in diseases where no medicine was given, were regarded as models of treatment worthy of imitation. But *this was a great error.* The pitiable and highly imperfect efforts of the vital force to relieve itself in acute diseases is a spectacle that should excite our compassion, and command the aid of all the powers of our rational mind, to terminate the self-inflicted torture by a real cure. If nature is unable to cure homœopathically a disease already existing in the organism, by the production of another fresh malady *similar* to it (§§ 43-46), which very rarely lies in her power (§ 50), and if to the organism alone is left the task of overcoming, by its own forces without external aid, a disease newly contracted (in cases of chronic miasms its power of resistance is quite inefficacious), we then witness nought but painful, often dangerous, efforts of nature to save the individual at whatever cost, which often terminate in extinction of the earthly existence, in death.

Little as we mortals know of the operations that take place in the interior economy in health—which must be hidden from us as certainly as they are patent to the eye of the all-seeing Creator and Preserver of his creatures—just as little can we perceive the operations that go on in the interior in disturbed conditions of life, in diseases. The internal operations in diseases are manifested only by the visible changes, the sufferings and the symptoms, whereby alone our life betrays the inward disturbance; so that in no given case can we ascertain which of the morbid symptoms are caused by the primary action of the morbific agent, which by the reaction of the vital force for its own relief.

in the slighter cases of acute disease; they merely imitated the unreasoning life-preserving power when left to itself in diseases, which entirely dependent as it is upon the organic laws of the body, is only capable of acting in conformity with these laws and is not guided by reason and reflection—they copied nature, which cannot, like an intelligent surgeon, bring together the gaping lips of a wound and by their union effect a cure; which knows not how to straighten and adjust the broken ends of a bone

---

Both are inextricably mixed up together before our eyes, and only present to us an outwardly reflected picture of the entire internal malady, for the fruitless efforts of unassisted vitality to terminate the sufferings are themselves sufferings of the whole organism. Hence, even in those evacuations termed *crises,* which nature generally produces at the termination of diseases which run a rapid course, there is frequently more of suffering than of efficacious relief.

What the vital force does in these so-called crises, and *how* it does it, remains a mystery to us, like all the internal operations of the organic vital economy. One thing, however, is certain: that in all these efforts *more or less of the affected parts are sacrificed and destroyed* in order to save the rest. These self-aiding operations of the vital force for the removal of an acute disease, performed only in obedience to the laws of organic life and not guided by the reflection of an intellect, are mostly but a species of allopathy; in order to relieve the primarily affected organ by a crisis, an increased, often violent, activity is excited in the excretory organs, to draw away the disease from the former to the latter; there ensue vomitings, purgings, diuresis, diaphoresis, abscesses, etc., in order, by this irritation of distant parts, to effect a sort of derivation from the primarily diseased part, and the dynamically affected nervous power seems to unload itself in the material product.

lying far apart and exuding much (often an excess of) new osseous matter; which cannot put a ligature on a wounded artery, but in its energy causes the patient to bleed to death; which does not understand how to replace a dislocated shoulder, but by the swelling it occasions round about it soon presents an obstacle to reduction; which in order to remove a foreign body from the cornea, destroys the whole eye by suppuration; which, with all its efforts can only liberate a strangulated hernia by gangrene of the bowel and death; and which, by the metaschematisms it produces in dynamic diseases, often renders them much worse than they were originally. But more, *this irrational vital force receives into our body, without hesitation,* the greatest plagues of our terrestrial existence, the spark that kindles the countless diseases beneath which tortured mankind has groaned for hundreds and thousands of year, the chronic miasms—psora, syphilis, sycosis—not one of which can it diminish in the slightest degree far less expel single-handed from the organism; on the contrary, it allows them to rankle therein

---

It is only by the destruction and sacrifice of a portion of the organism itself that unaided nature can save the patient in acute diseases, and, if death do not ensue, restore, though only slowly and imperfectly, the harmony of life—health.

The great weakness of the parts which had been exposed to the disease, and even of the whole body, the emaciation, etc., remaining after spontaneous cures, are convincing proofs of this.

In short, the whole operation of the self-aiding power of the organism when attacked by diseases displays to the observer nothing but suffering—nothing that he could or ought to imitate if he wishes to cure disease in a truly artistic manner.

until often after a long life of misery, death at last closes the eyes of the sufferer.

In such an important affair as that of healing, which demands so much intelligence, reflection and judgment, how could the old school, which arrogates to itself the title of rational, choose as its best instructor, as its guide to be blindly followed, the unintelligent vital force, inconsiderately copy its indirect and revolutionary operations in diseases, imagining these to be the *non plus ultra,* the best conceivable, when that greatest gift of God, reflective reason and unfettered judgment, was given us to enable us infinitely to surpass it in salutary help to suffering humanity?

When the old school practitioners, thoughtlessly imitating the crude, senseless, automatic vital energy with their counter-irritant and derivative methods of treatment—by far their most usual plans—attack innocent parts and organs of the body, either inflicting on them excruciating pains, or as is most frequently done, compelling them to perform evacuations whereby strength and fluids are wasted, their object is to direct the morbid vital action in the primarily affected parts away to those artificially attacked, and thus to effect the cure of the natural disease indirectly, *by the production of a disease much greater in intensity and of quite a different kind,* in the healthy parts of the body, consequently by a circuitous way, at the cost of much loss of strength, and usually of great suffering to the patient.[19]

---

[19] Daily experience shows the sad effects of this manœuvre in chronic diseases. *Anything but a cure is effected.* Who would

The disease, if it be acute, and consequently naturally of but short duration, may certainly disappear, even during these heterogeneous attacks on distant and dissimilar parts—but it is not cured. There is nothing that can merit the honorable name of *cure* in this revolutionary treatment, which has no direct, immediate, pathological relation to the tissues primarily affected. Often indeed, without these serious attacks on the rest of the organism, would the acute disease have ceased of itself, sooner most likely, with fewer subsequent sufferings and less sacrifice of strength. But neither the mode of operation of the crude natural forces, nor the allopathic copy of that, can for a moment be compared to the dynamic (homœopathic) treatment, which sustains the strength, while it extinguishes the disease in a direct and rapid manner.

---

ever call that a victory if, in place of attacking the enemy in front in a hand-to-hand fight, and by his destruction terminating at once his hostile assaults, we should, in a cowardly manner and behind his back, lay an embargo on everything, cut off his supplies, burn down everything for a great way round him? By so doing we would at length deprive him of all courage to resist, but our object is not gained, the enemy is far from being destroyed,—he is still there, and when he can again procure provisions and supplies, he once more rears his head, more exasperated than before—the enemy, I repeat, is far from being destroyed, but the poor innocent country is so completely ruined that it will be long before it can recover itself. In like manner acts allopathy in chronic diseases, when, by its indirect attacks on innocent parts at a distance from the seat of the disease, instead of effecting a cure, it destroys the organism. Such is the result of its hurtful operations!

In far the greatest number of cases of disease, however—I mean those of a chronic nature—these perturbing, debilitating, indirect modes of treatment of the old school are scarcely ever of the slightest use. They suspend for a few days only, some troublesome symptom or other, which, however, returns when the system has become accustomed to the distant irritation, and the disease recurs worse than before, because by the antagonistic pains[20] and the injudicious evacuations the vital powers have been depressed.

Whilst most physicians of the old school, *imitating in a general manner* the efforts of crude, unaided nature for its own relief, carried out in their practice these derivations of merely hypothetical utility, just as they judged expedient (guided by some imaginary indication), others, aiming at a higher object, undertook *designedly to promote the efforts of the vital force to aid itself by evacuations and antagonistic metastases, as seen in diseases,* and by way of lending it a helping hand, to increase still more these derivations and evacuations; and they believed that by this hurtful procedure they were acting *duce natura,* and might justly claim the title of *minister naturæ.*

---

[20] What good results have ever ensued from those fœtid artificial ulcers, so much in vogue, called issues? If even during the first week or two, whilst they still cause pain, they appear somewhat to check by antagonism a chronic disease, yet by and by, when the body has become accustomed to the pain, they have *no* other effect than that of weakening the patient and giving still greater scope to the chronic affection. Or does anyone imagine, in this nineteenth century, that they serve as an outlet for the escape of the *materia peccans?* It almost appears as if this were the case!

As the evacuations effected by the natural powers of the patient in chronic diseases are not infrequently the precursors of alleviations—though only of a temporary character—of troublesome symptoms, violent pains, paralyses, spasms, etc., so the old school imagined these derivations to be the true way of curing diseases, and endeavored to promote, maintain and even increase such evacuations. But they did not perceive that all these evacuations and excretions (pseudo-crises) produced by nature when left to herself were, in chronic diseases, only palliative, transient alleviations which, far from contributing to a real cure, on the contrary, rather aggravate the original, internal dyscrasia, by the waste of strength and juices they occasioned. No one ever saw a chronic patient recover his health permanently by such efforts of crude nature, nor any chronic disease cured by such evacuations effected by the organism.[21] On the contrary, in such cases the original dyscrasia is always perceptibly aggravated, after alleviations, whose duration always becomes shorter and shorter; the bad attacks recur more frequently and more severely in spite of the continuation of the evacuations. In like manner, on the occurrence of symptoms excited by an internal chronic affection that threaten to destroy life, when nature left to its own resources, cannot help herself in any other way than by the production of external local symptoms, in order to avert the danger from parts indispensable to life and direct it to tissues of less vital importance (metastasis), these operations of the energetic but unintelligent, unreasoning and improvident

---

[21] Equally inefficacious are those produced artificially.

vital force conduce to anything but genuine relief or recovery; they only silence in a palliative manner, for a short time, the dangerous internal affection at the cost of a large portion of the humours and of the strength, without diminishing the original disease by a hair's breadth; they can, at the most, only retard the fatal termination which is inevitable without true homœopathic treatment.

The allopathy of the old school not only greatly overrated these efforts of the crude automatic power of nature, but completely misjudged them, falsely considered them to be truly curative, and endeavored to increase and promote them, vainly imagining that thereby they might perhaps succeed in annihilating and radically curing the whole disease. When, in chronic diseases, the vital force seemed to silence this or that troublesome symptom of the internal affection by the production, for example, of some humid cutaneous eruption, then the servant of the crude power of nature (*minister naturæ*) applied to the discharging surface a cantharides plaster or an exutory (mezereum), in order, *duce natura,* to draw still more moisture from the skin, and thus to promote and to assist nature's object—the cure (by the removal of the morbific matter from the body?) ; but when the effect of the remedy was too violent, the eczema already of long standing, and the system too irritable, he increased the external affection to a great degree without the slightest advantage, to the original disease, and aggravated the pains, which deprived the patient of sleep and depressed his strength (and sometimes even developed a malignant febrile erysipelas) ; or if the effect upon the local affection (still recent, perhaps) was of milder character, he thereby repelled from its seat, by a species of ill-applied external homœopathy, the local symptom which had been established by nature on the skin for the relief of the internal disease, thus renewing the more dangerous internal malady, and by this repulsion of the local symptom compelling the vital force to effect a transference of a worse form of morbid action to other and more important parts, the patient became affected with dangerous ophthalmia, or deafness, or spasms of the stomach, or epileptic convulsions, or attacks of asthma or apoplexy, or mental derangement, etc., in place of the repelled local disease.[22]

When the diseased natural force propelled blood into the veins of the rectum or anus (blind hæmorrhoids), the *minister naturæ,* under the same delusive idea of assisting the vital force in its curative efforts, applied leeches, often in large numbers, in order to give an outlet to the blood there—with but brief, often scarcely noteworthy, relief, but thereby weakening the body and occasioning still greater congestions in those parts, without the slightest diminution of the original disease.

In almost all cases in which the diseased vital force endeavored to subdue the violence of a dangerous internal malady by evacuating blood by means of vomiting, coughing, etc., the old school physician, *duce natura,* made haste to assist these supposed salutary efforts of nature, and performed a copious venesection, which was invari-

---

[22] Natural effects of the repulsion of these local symptoms—effects that are often regarded by the allopathic physician as fresh diseases of quite a different kind.

ably productive of injurious consequences and palpable weakening of the body.

In cases of frequently occurring chronic nausea, he produced, with the view of furthering the intentions of nature, copious evacuations of the stomach, by means of powerful emetics—never with a good result, often with bad, not infrequently dangerous and even fatal consequences.

The vital force, in order to relieve the internal malady, sometimes produces indolent enlargements of the external glands, and he thinks to forward the intentions of nature, in his assumed character of her servant, when, by the use of all sorts of heating embrocations and plasters, he causes them to inflame, so that, when the abscess is ripe, he may incise it and let out the bad morbific matter (?). Experience has shown, hundreds of times, that lasting evil almost invariably results from such a plan.

And having often noticed slight amelioration of the severe symptoms of chronic diseases to result from spontaneous night sweats or frequent liquid stools, he imagines himself bound to obey these hints of nature (*duce natura*), and to promote them, by instituting and maintaining a complete course of sweating treatment or by the employment of so-called gentle laxatives for years, in order to promote and increase these efforts of nature (of the vital force of the unintelligent organism), which he thinks tend to the cure of the whole chronic affection, and thus to free the patient more speedily and certainly from his disease (the matter of his disease?).

But he thereby always produces quite the contrary result: aggravation of the original disease.

5

In conformity with this preconceived but unfounded idea, the old school physician goes on thus promoting[23] the efforts of the diseased vital force and increasing those derivations and evacuations in the patient which *never* lead to the desired end, but are *always* disastrous, without being aware that all the local affections, evacuations, and seemingly derivative efforts, set up and continued by the unintelligent vital force when left to its own resources, for

---

[23] In direct opposition to this treatment, the old school not infrequently indulged themselves in the very reverse of this: thus, when the efforts of the vital force for the relief of the internal disease by evacuations and the production of local symptoms on the exterior of the body became troublesome, they capriciously suppressed them by their *repercutients* and *repellents;* they subdued chronic pains, sleeplessness and diarrhœa of long standing by doses of opium pushed to a dangerous extent; vomitings by effervescent saline draughts; fœtid perspiration of the feet by cold footbaths and astringent applications; eruptions on the skin by preparations of lead and zinc; they checked uterine hæmorrhage by injections of vinegar; colliquative perspiration by alum; nocturnal seminal emissions by the free use of camphor; frequent attacks of flushes of heat in the body and face by nitre, vegetable acids and sulphuric acid; bleeding of the nose by plugging the nostrils with dossils of lint soaked in alcohol or astringent fluids; they dried up discharging ulcers on the legs, established by the vital power for the relief of great internal suffering, with the oxides of lead and zinc, etc., with what sad results experience has shown in thousands of cases.

With tongue and with pen the old school physician brags that he is a rational practitioner, and that he investigates the cause of the disease so as always to make radical cures; but behold, his treatment is directed, in these cases, against a single symptom only, and always with injurious consequences to his patient.

the relief of the original chronic disease, are actually the disease itself, the phenomena of the whole disease, for the totality of which, properly speaking, the only efficacious remedy, and the one, moreover, that will act in the most direct manner, is a homœopathic medicine, chosen on account of its similarity of action.

As everything that crude nature does to relieve itself in diseases, in those of an acute, but especially those of a chronic kind, is extremely imperfect and even *actual disease*, it may easily be conceived that the promotion by artificial means of this imperfection and disease must do still more harm; at least, it cannot improve the efforts of nature for its own relief, even in acute diseases, because medical art is not in a condition to follow the hidden paths by which the vital force effects its crises, but attempts to produce them from without, by violent means, which are still less beneficial than what the instinctive vital force left to its own resources does, but on the other hand are more perturbing and debilitating. For even the incomplete amelioration resulting from the natural derivations and crises cannot be obtained in a similar manner by allopathy; with all its endeavors it cannot procure anything like even that pitiful relief the vital force left to itself is able to afford.

It has been attempted to produce, by means of scarifying instruments, a bleeding at the nose, in imitation of that sometimes occurring naturally, in order to mitigate, for example, the attacks of a chronic headache. By this means a large quantity of blood could be made to flow from the nostrils and weaken the patient, but the relief afforded was either nil, or much less than the instinctive vital force would procure at another time, when, of its own accord, it would cause but a few drops to flow.

A so-called critical perspiration or diarrhœa, produced by the ever active vital force after a sudden indisposition, excited by anger, fright, a sprain or a chill, will be much more successful, at least for the time, in relieving the acute disease, than all the sudorific or purgative drugs in the pharmacopœia, which only make the patient worse, as daily experience shows.

But the vital force, which of itself can only act according to the physical constitution of our organism, and is not guided by reason, knowledge and reflection, was not given to man to be regarded as the best possible curative agent to restore those lamentable deviations from health to the normal condition, and still less that physicians should slavishly imitate its imperfect morbid efforts (to free itself from disease), and that with operations incontestably more inappropriate and severe than its own, and thereby conveniently spare themselves the expenditure of reasoning, reflection and judgment requisite for the discovery and for the practice of the noblest of human arts — the true healing art — while they allege their bad copy of the spontaneous efforts of doubtful utility made by the crude natural force for its relief, to be the healing art, *the rational healing art!*

What sensible man would imitate the efforts of the organism for its own preservation? These efforts are in reality the disease itself, and the morbidly affected vital force is the producer of the visible disease! It must, therefore, necessarily follow that all artificial imitation, and likewise the suppression of these efforts, must either increase the disease or render it dangerous by their suppression, and both of these allopathy does; these are its pernicious operations which it alleges to be the healing art, the rational healing art!

No! that exquisite power innate in the human being, designed to direct in the most perfect manner the operations of life *while it is in health,* equally present in all parts of the organism, in the fibres of sensibility as well as in those of irritability, the unwearying spring of all the normal natural functions of the body, was not created for the purpose of affording itself aid in diseases, not for the purpose of exercising a healing art worthy of imitation. *No! the true healing art is that reflective work, the attribute of the higher powers of human intellect, of unfettered judgment and of reason selecting and determining on principle in order to effect an alteration in the instinctive, irrational and unintelligent, but energetic automatic vital force, when it has been diverted by disease into abnormal action, and by means of a similar affection developed by a homœopathically chosen remedy, to excite in it a medicinal disease somewhat greater in degree, so that the natural morbid affection can no longer act upon the vital force, which thus, freed from the natural disease, has now only the similar, somewhat stronger, medicinal morbid affection to contend with, against which it now directs its whole energy and which it soon overpowers, whereby the vital force is liberated and enabled to return to the normal standard of health and to its proper function, "the maintenance of the life and health of the organism," without having suffered, during this change, any painful or debilitating attacks. Homœopathy teaches us how to effect this.*

Under the methods of treatment of the old school I
have just detailed, no small number of patients certainly
got rid of their diseases but not of those of a chronic
(non-venereal) character; only such as were acute and
unattended with danger; and even these they were only
freed from by such circuitous and tedious ways, and
often so incompletely, that the results of the treatment
could never be termed cures effected by a gentle art.
Acute diseases of a not very dangerous kind were, by
venesections or suppression of one of the chief symptoms
through the instrumentality of an enantiopathic palliative
remedy (*contraria contrariis*), kept under, or by means of
counter-irritant and derivative (antagonistic and revul-
sive) remedies, applied to other than the diseased spots,
suspended, until the natural time for the duration of the
short malady had expired. These methods were, consequently, indirect, and attended with loss of strength and
humours, so much so that in patients so treated the
greatest and most important measures for the complete
removal of the disease and for the restoration of the lost
strength and humours remained to be performed by
Nature herself—by the life-preserving power which, besides the removal of the natural acute disease, had also
to combat the effects of improper treatment, and thus it
was able, in cases unattended by danger, gradually to
restore the normal relation of the functions by means of
its own energy, but often in a tedious, imperfect and
painful manner.

It remains a very doubtful question whether the
natural process of recovery in acute diseases is really at
all shortened or facilitated by this interference of the old

school, as the latter cannot act otherwise than the vital force, namely, indirectly; but its derivative and counter-irritant treatment is much more injurious and much more debilitating.

The old school has yet another method of treatment, which is termed the *stimulating and strengthening* system[24] (by *excitantia, nervina, tonica, confortantia, roborantia*). It is astonishing how it can boast of this method.

Has it ever succeeded in removing the physical weakness so often engendered and kept up or increased by a chronic disease with its prescriptions of etheric Rhine-wine or fiery Tokay? The strength gradually sank under this treatment, and all the lower, the greater the quantity of wine the patient was persuaded to drink, because the source of weakness, the chronic disease, was not cured by it, because artificial stimulation is followed by relaxation in the reaction of the vital force.

Or did its cinchona bark, or its *amara,* so misunderstood, so multifarious in their modes of action, and productive of quite different kinds of injury, give strength in these frequently occurring cases? Did not these vegetable substances, said to be tonic and strengthening under all circumstances, as also the preparations of iron, often add to the old disease new sufferings, by virtue of their peculiar pathogenetic effects, without relieving the weakness proceeding from an unknown disease of long standing?

---

[24] It is, properly speaking, enantiopathic, and I shall again refer to it in the text of the *Organon* (§ 59).

Has any one ever succeeded in diminishing in the very least the duration of the incipient paralysis of an arm or a leg, so often arising from a chronic dyscrasia, by means of the so-called *unguenta nervina* or any other spirituous or balsamic embrocations, without curing the dyscrasia itself. Or have electric or galvanic shocks ever been attended with any other result in such cases, than a gradually increasing, and finally absolute, paralysis, and extinction of all muscular and nervous irritability in the affected limbs?[25]

Did not the renowned *excitantia* and *aphrodisiaca,* ambergris, lacerta scincus, cantharides tincture, truffles, cardamoms, cinnamon and vanilla invariably bring about complete impotence when used for the purpose of restoring the gradually declining sexual power (which always depended on an unobserved chronic miasm)?

How can credit be taken for the production of a stimulation and invigoration of but a few hours' duration, when the result that must follow and which is permanent —according to the laws of all palliative action—is a directly opposite state, the rendering of the disease incurable?

The little good that the *excitantia* and *roborantia* did for recovery from acute diseases (treated according to the

---

[25] Those affected with hardness of hearing were relieved by moderate shocks from the voltaic pile of the apothecary of Jever only for a few hours—these moderate shocks soon lost their power. In order to produce the same result he had to make them stronger; until these stronger shocks had no effect; the very strongest would then at first excite the patients' hearing for a short time, but at length left them quite deaf.

old method) was a thousand times outweighed by their ill effects in chronic maladies.

When physicians of the old school do not know what to do in a chronic disease, they treat it blindly with their so-called *alterative* remedies (*alterantia*) ; among which the horrible *mercurialia* (calomel, corrosive sublimate and mercurial ointment) occupy the foremost place—which they allow to act in such large quantities and for so long a time on the diseased body (in non-venereal diseases!) that at last the health is by their destructive effects completely undermined. They thus certainly produce great alterations, but invariably such as are not beneficial, and they always utterly ruin the health by their improper administration of this excessively injurious metal.

When they prescribe, in large doses, *cinchona bark* (which, as a homœopathic febrifuge, is only specific in true marsh ague, accompanied with psora), for all epidemic intermittent fevers, which are often distributed over large tracts of country, the old school practitioners palpably manifest their stupidity, for these diseases assume a different character almost every year and hence demand for their cure, almost always, a different homœopathic remedy, by means of one or a few very small doses of which they may always be radically cured in a few days. Now, because these epidemic fevers have periodical attacks (*typus*) and the adherents of the old school see nothing in all intermittent fevers, but their *typus* [periodicity], and neither know nor care to know any other febrifuge but cinchona, these routine practitioners imagine if they can but suppress the *typus* of the epidemic intermittent fever with enormous doses of cinchona and its costly alkaloid, quinine (an event which the unintelli-

gent, but, in this instance, more sensible vital force endeavors to prevent often for months), that they have
cured this epidemic ague. But the deluded patient, after
such a suppression of the periodicity (*typus*) of his fever,
invariably becomes worse than he was during the fever
itself; with sallow complexion, dyspnœa, constriction in
the hypochondria, disordered bowels, unhealthy appetite,
broken sleep, feeble and desponding, often with great
swelling of the legs, of the abdomen and even of the
face and hands, he creeps out of the hospital, *dismissed
as cured,* and long years of homœopathic treatment are
not infrequently required, merely to rescue from death,
let alone to cure and restore to health, such a profoundly
injured (cured?), artificially cachectic patient.

The old school is happy when it can convert the dull
stupor that occurs in typhus fevers, by means of *valerian,*
which in this case acts antipathically, into a kind of liveliness of a few hours' duration; but as this does not continue, and to force a repetition of the animation ever
increasing doses of valerian are requisite, it is not long
before the largest doses cease to have the desired effect.
But as this palliative is only stimulant in its primary
action, in its after effects the vital force is paralysed, and
such a patient is certain of a speedy death from this
rational treatment of the old school; none can escape.
And yet the adherents of this routine art could not perceive that by these proceedings they most certainly killed
their patients; they ascribed the death to the malignancy
of the disease.

A palliative of a still more horrible character for chronic
patients is the *digitalis purpurea,* with which the old school
practitioners imagine they do such excellent service, when

by means of it, they compel the quick, irritated pulse in chronic diseases (purely symptomatic!) to become slower. True it is that this dreadful remedy, which is in such cases employed enantiopathically, strikingly diminishes the frequency of the quick, irritated pulse, and greatly reduces the number of the arterial pulsations, *for a few hours after the first dose;* but the pulse soon becomes more rapid than before. In order again to diminish in some degree its frequency the dose is increased, and it has the effect, but for a still shorter period, until even these and still larger palliative doses cease to reduce the pulse, which at length, in the secondary action of the foxglove which can no longer be restrained, becomes much more rapid than it was before the use of this drug,—it then becomes *uncountable;* sleep, appetite and strength are lost—death is imminent; *not one of the patients so treated escapes alive,* unless to be a prey to incurable insanity![26]

Such was the treatment pursued by the allopathist. The patients, therefore, *were obliged* to yield to the sad necessity, because they could obtain no better aid from other allopathists, who had gained their knowledge from the same deceitful books.

As the fundamental cause of chronic (non-venereal) diseases, together with the remedies for them, remained

---

[26] And yet Hufeland, the chief of this old school (v. *Homöo-pathie,* p. 22), extols with much satisfaction the employment of *digitalis* in such cases, in these words: "None will deny" (experience invariably does so!) "that too great rapidity of the circulation can be *removed* (?) by *digitalis.*" Permanently removed? and by a heroic enantiopathic remedy? Poor Hufeland!

unknown to these practitioners, who vainly boasted of
their causal medication and of their diagnosis being directed to the investigation of the *genesis* of diseases[27];
how could they hope to cure the immense numbers of
chronic diseases by their indirect treatments, which were
but hurtful imitations of the unintelligent vital force for
its own relief, that never were intended to be models for
practice?

The presumed character of the affection they regarded
as the cause of the disease, and hence they directed their
pretended causal treatment against spasm, inflammation
(plethora), fever, general and partial debility, mucus,
putridity, obstructions, etc., which they thought to remove
by means of their antispasmodic, antiphlogistic, tonic,
stimulant, antiseptic, dissolvent, resolvent, derivative,
evacuant, antagonistic remedies (of which they only possessed a superficial knowledge).

But from such general indications really serviceable
medicines could not be discovered, most assuredly not in
the materia medica of the old school, which, as I have
elsewhere shown,[28] is founded mainly on conjecture and
false deductions *ab usu in morbis,* mixed up with false-
hood and fraud.

---

[27] Which Hufeland in his pamphlet, *Die Homöopathie,* page 20,
makes a futile attempt to appropriate for his old psuedo-art. For
since, as is well known, previous to the appearance of my book
(*Chronic Diseases*), the 2500-years-old allopathy knew nothing
about the source of most chronic diseases (psora), must it not
have attributed a false source (*genesis*) to such maladies?

[28] See essay in the first volume of the *Materia Medica Pura*
(English edit.), "Sources of the Common Materia Medica."

With equal rashness they attacked those still more hypothetical so-called indications — deficiency or excess of oxygen, nitrogen, carbon, or hydrogen in the fluids, exaltation or diminution of the irritability, sensibility and reproduction, derangements of the arterial, venous and capillary systems, asthenia, etc., without knowing a single remedy for effecting objects so visionary. All this was pure ostentation. It was a mode of treatment that did no good to the patients.

But all semblance of appropriate treatment of diseases was completely lost by a practice, introduced in the earliest times, *and even made into a rule:* I mean the *mixture in a prescription* of various medicinal substances, whose real action was, almost without an exception, unknown, and which, without any one exception, invariably differed so much among each other. One medicine (the sphere of whose medicinal effects was unknown) was placed foremost, as the principal remedy (*basis*), and was designed to subdue what the physician deemed the chief character of the disease, to this was added some other drug (equally unknown as regards the sphere of its medicinal action) for the removal of some accessory symptom, or to strengthen the action of the first (*adjuvans*); and besides these, yet another (likewise unknown as to the sphere of its medicinal powers), a pretended corrective remedy (*corrigens*); these were all *mixed together* (boiled, infused)—and along with them, some medicinal syrup, or distilled medicinal water, also with different properties, would be included in the formula, and it was supposed that each of the ingredients of this mixture would perform, in the diseased body, the part allotted to it by the prescriber's imagination, with-

out suffering itself to be disturbed or led astray by
the other things mixed up along with it; which, however, could not in reason be expected. One ingredient
suspended wholly or partially the action of another, or
communicated to it and to the others a mode of action
and operation not anticipated nor conjecturable, so that
it was *impossible* the expected effect could be obtained;
there *frequently* occurred a *new morbid derangement,*
which, from the incomprehensible changes imparted to
substances by their admixture, was not and could not
have been foreseen, which escaped observation amid the
tumultuous symptoms of the disease, and which became
permanent from a lengthened employment of the prescription—accordingly an artificial disease was added to
and complicated the original disease, causing an aggravation of the latter—or if the prescription were not often
repeated, but superseded by one or more new prescriptions, composed of other ingredients, given in rapid succession, then the *very least* that could happen was *a
farther depression of the strength,* for the substances
administered in that way neither had, nor could have
had, any direct pathological relation to the original
malady, but only attacked, in a useless and injurious
manner, parts that were least implicated in the disease.

The mixture of several medicines, even if the effects
of each single medicine on the human body were accurately known (—the prescription writer, however, often
knows not the thousandth part of their effects—), the
association, in one prescription, of several such ingredients, I repeat, many of which are themselves of a very
compound nature, and the peculiar action of any one of
which is as good as unknown, although in reality it al-

ways differs greatly from that of the others, and the administration of this incomprehensible mixture to the patient in large and frequently repeated doses, in order therewith to obtain some purposed, certain, curative effect, is a piece of folly repugnant to every reflecting and unprejudiced person.[29]

---

[29] The absurdity of medicinal mixtures was perceived even by adherents of the old school of medicine, although they still continued to follow this slovenly plan in their own practice, contrary to their convictions. Thus Marcus Herz (in *Hufeland's Journal*, ii, p. 33) reveals the pricks of his conscience in the following words: "When we wish to remove the inflammatory state, we do not employ either nitre or sal-ammoniac or vegetable acids alone, but we usually mix several, and often but too many, so-called anti-phlogistics together, or give them in the same case in close succession. If we have to combat putridity, we are not content to look for the attainment of our object from the administrations of large doses of one of the known antiseptic medicines, such as cinchona bark, mineral acids, arnica, serpentaria, etc., alone; we prefer associating several of them together, and count upon their community of action; or from our uncertainty as to whose action is the most suitable for the case in question, we throw together a number of different substances, and almost leave it to chance to effect the end we have in view, by means of one of them. Thus we seldom excite perspiration, purify the blood (?), overcome obstructions (?), promote expectoration, or even evacuate the primæ viæ, by a single remedy; our prescriptions for these objects are always composite, almost never simple and pure, *consequently neither are our observations in reference to the actions of each individual substance contained in them.* To be sure, we learnedly institute certain grades of rank among the remedies in our formulas; on the one to which we particularly commission the action, we confer the title of *base* (basis), the others we call *helpers, supporters* (adjuvantia), *correctives* (cor-

The result naturally belies every expectation that had been formed. There certainly ensue changes and results, but none of an appropriate character, none beneficial— all injurious, destructive!

I should like to see any one who would call the purblind inroads of such prescriptions on the diseased human body a *cure!*

It is only by guiding what still remains of the vital principle in the patient to the proper performance of its functions, by means of a suitable medicine, that a cure can be expected, but not by enervating the body to death, *secundum artem;* and yet the old school knows not what **else** to do with patients suffering from chronic diseases, **than** to attack the sufferers with drugs that do nothing

---

rigentia), etc. But this classification is evidently almost entirely arbitrary. The *helpers* and *supporters* have just as much part in the whole action as the *chief ingredient,* although, from want of a standard of measurement, we are unable to determine the degree of their participation in the result. In like manner the influence of the *correctives* on the powers of the other ingredients cannot be quite indifferent; they must increase or diminish them, or give them quite another direction; and hence we must always regard the salutary (?) change which we effect, by means of such a prescription, as the result of all its ingredients collectively, and *we can never obtain from its action a pure experience of the individual efficacy of any single ingredient of which it is composed. In fact, our knowledge of what is essential to be known respecting all our remedies, as also respecting the perhaps hundred-fold relationship among each other into which they enter when combined, is far too little to be relied upon to enable us to tell with certainty the degree and extent of the action of a substance, seemingly ever so unimportant, when introduced into the human body in combination with other substances."*

but torture them, waste their strength and fluids, and shorten their lives! Can it be said to save whilst it destroys? Does it deserve any other name than that of a *mischievous* [non-healing] *art?* It acts, *lege artis,* in the most inappropriate manner, and it does (it would almost seem *purposely*) ἀλλοῖα that is to say, the very opposite of what it should do. Can it be commended? Can it be any longer tolerated?

In recent times the old school practitioners have quite surpassed themselves in their cruelty towards their sick fellow-creatures, and in the unsuitableness of their operations, as every unprejudiced observer must admit, and as even physicians of their own school have been forced, by the pricks of their conscience (like Krüger Hansen), to confess before the world.

It was high time for the wise and benevolent Creator and Preserver of mankind to put a stop to these abominations, to command a cessation of these tortures, and to reveal a healing art the very opposite of all this, which should not waste the vital juices and powers by emetics, perennial scourings out of the bowels, warm baths, diaphoretics or salivation; nor shed the life's blood, nor torment and weaken with painful appliances; nor, in place of curing patients, suffering from diseases, render them incurable by the addition of new, chronic medicinal maladies by means of the prolonged use of wrong, powerful medicines of unknown properties; nor yoke the horse behind the cart, by giving strong palliatives, according to the old favorite axiom, *contraria contrariis curentur;* nor, in short, in place of lending the patient aid, to guide him in the way to death, as is done by the merciless routine practitioner;—but which, on the contrary, should spare the patient's strength as much as possible, and should, rapidly and mildly, effect an unalloyed and permanent cure, and restore to health by means of smallest doses of few simple medicines carefully selected according to their proved effects, by the only therapeutic law conformable to nature: *similia similibus curentur*. It was high time that he should permit the discovery of homœopathy.

By observation, reflection and experience, I discovered that, contrary to the old allopathic method, the true, the proper, the best mode of treatment is contained in the maxim: *To cure mildly, rapidly, certainly, and permanently, choose, in every case of disease, a medicine which can itself produce an affection similar* (ὅμοιον πάθος) *to that sought to be cured!*

Hitherto no one has ever *taught* this homœopathic mode of cure, no one has *carried it out in practice*. But if the truth is only to be found in this method, as I can prove it to be, we might expect that, even though it remained *unperceived* for thousands of years, distinct traces of it would yet be discovered in every age.[80]

And such is the fact. In all ages, the patients *who have been really, rapidly, permanently and obviously*

---

[80] For truth is co-eternal with the all-wise, benevolent Deity. It may long escape the observation of man, until the time foreordained by Providence arrives, when its rays shall irresistibly break through the clouds of prejudice and usher in the dawn of a day which shall shine with a bright and inextinguishable light for the weal of the human race.

cured by medicines, and who did not merely *recover* by some fortuitous circumstance, or by the acute disease having run its allotted course, or by the powers of the system having, in the course of time, gradually attained the preponderance, under allopathic and antagonistic treatment—for being cured in a direct manner differs vastly from recovering in an indirect manner—such patients have been cured solely (although without the knowledge of the physician) by means of a (homœopathic) medicine which possessed the power of producing a similar morbid state.

Even in *real* cures by means of mixtures of medicines —which were excessively rare—it will be found that the remedy whose action predominated was always of a homœopathic character.

But this is observed much more strikingly in cases where physicians sometimes effected a rapid cure with one simple medicinal substance, contrary to the usual custom, that admitted of none but mixtures of medicines in the form of a prescription. There we see, to our astonishment, that this always occurred by means of a medicine that is *itself* capable of producing an affection similar to the case of disease, although the physicians themselves knew not what they were doing, and acted in forgetfulness of the contrary doctrines of their own school. They prescribed a medicine the very reverse of that which they should have employed according to the traditional therapeutics, and it was *only in consequence of so doing* that the patients were rapidly cured.

If we deduct the cases in which the specific remedy for a disease of never varying character has been made known to physicians of the ordinary school (not by their

own investigation, but) *by the empirical practice of the
common people,* wherewith they are enabled to effect a
direct cure, as for instance, of the venereal chancrous
disease with mercury; of the morbid state resulting from
contusions with arnica; of marsh ague with cinchona
bark; of recent cases of itch with flowers of sulphur, etc.
—if we deduct these, we find, that without almost *any*
exception, all the other treatment of the old school physician, in chronic diseases, consists in debilitating, teasing
and tormenting the already afflicted patient, to the
aggravation of his disease and to his destruction, with a
great display of dignified gravity on the part of the
doctor and at a ruinous expense to the patient.

Blind experience sometimes led them to a homœopathic
mode of treatment,[31] and yet they did not perceive the

---

[31] Thus they imagined they could drive out through the skin
the sudatory matter which they believed to stagnate there after a
chill, if they gave the patient to drink, during the cold stage of
the catarrhal fever, an infusion of elder flowers, which is capable
of removing such a fever and curing the patient by its peculiar
similarity of action (homœopathically), and this it does most
promptly and effectually, without causing perspiration, if but a
small quantity of this infusion, and nothing else, be taken. To
hard, acute swellings, in which the excessive violence of the inflammation prevents their suppuration and causes intolerable pains,
they apply very warm poultices, frequently renewed, and behold!
the inflammation and the pains diminish rapidly, while the abscess is rapidly formed, as is known by the yellowish shining eleva-
tion and the perceptible softening. In this case they imagine
that the hardness has been softened by the *moisture* of the poultice, whereas it is chiefly by the greater heat of the poultices that
the excess of inflammation has been homœopathically subdued, and
the rapid suppuration been enabled to take place.—Why do they

law of nature in obedience to which cures so effected did and must ensue.

Hence it is highly important, for the weal of mankind, to ascertain what really took place in these extremely rare but singularly salutary treatments. The answer we obtain to this question is of the utmost significance.

---

employ with benefit in many ophthalmiæ St. Yve's salve, the chief ingredient of which is red oxide of mercury, which can produce inflammation of the eyes, if anything can? Is it hard to see that they here act homœopathically?—Or why should a little parsley juice produce such evident relief in those cases (by no means rare), where there are anxious, often ineffectual, efforts to urinate in little children, and in ordinary gonorrhœa, which is well known by the very painful, frequent and almost ineffectual attempts to make water, if the fresh juice of this plant had not the power of causing, in healthy persons, a painful, almost fruitless, urging to urinate, consequently cures homœopathically? With the pimpernal root, which causes great secretion of mucus in the bronchia and fauces, they successfully combatted the so-called mucous angina—and quelled some kinds of metrorrhagia with the leaves of savine, which can itself cause metrorrhagia, without perceiving the homœopathic curative law. In cases of constipation from incarcerated hernia and in ileus many medical men found the constipating opium, in small doses, to be the most excellent and certain remedy, without having the most distant idea of the homœopathic therapeutic law exemplified in this case. They cured nonvenereal ulcers of the fauces with small doses of mercury, which is homœopathic to such states—stopped some diarrhœas with small doses of the purgative rhubarb—cured hydrophobia with belladonna, that causes a similar affection, and removed, as if by magic, the dangerous comatose state in acute fevers with a small dose of the heating, stupefying opium; and yet they abuse homœopathy, and persecute it with a fury that can only arise from the stings of an evil conscience in a heart incapable of improvement.

They were never performed in any other manner than by means of medicines of homœopathic power, that is to say, capable of producing a disease similar to the morbid state sought to be cured; the cures were effected rapidly and permanently by medicines, the medical prescribers of which made use of them as it were by accident, and even in opposition to the doctrines of all previous systems and therapeutics (often without rightly knowing what they were doing and why they did it), and thus, against their will, they practically confirmed the necessity of the only therapeutic law consonant to nature, that of homœopathy—a therapeutic law, which, despite the many facts and innumerable hints that pointed to it, no physicians of past epochs have exerted themselves to discover, blinded as they all have been by medical prejudices.

For even the domestic practice of the non-medical classes of the community endowed with sound observant faculties has many times proved this mode of treatment to be the surest, the most radical and the least fallacious in practice.

In recent cases of frost-bitten limbs frozen sour crout is applied or frictions of snow are used.[32]

---

[32] It is on such examples of domestic practice that Mr. M. Lux founds his so-called mode of cure by *identicals* and *idem,* which he calls *Isopathy,* which some eccentric-minded persons have already adopted as the *non plus ultra* of a therapeutic method, without knowing how they could carry it out.

But if we examine these instances attentively we find that they do not bear out these views.

The purely physical powers differ in the nature of their action on the living organism from those of a dynamic medicinal kind.

Heat or cold of the air that surrounds us, or of the water, or

The experienced cook holds his hand, which he has scalded, at a certain distance from the fire, and does not

---

of our food and drink, occasion (*as heat and cold*) *of themselves* no absolute injury to a healthy body; heat and cold are in their alternations essential to the maintenance of healthy life, consequently they are not of themselves medicine. Heat and cold, therefore, act as curative agents in affections of the body, not by virtue of their essential nature (not, therefore, as cold and heat *per se*, not as things hurtful in themselves, as are the drugs, rhubarb, china, etc., even in the smallest doses), but *only* by virtue of their greater or smaller *quantity*, that is, according to their degrees of temperature, just as (to take an example from purely physical powers) a great weight of lead will bruise my hand painfully, not by virtue of its essential nature as lead, for a thin plate of lead would not bruise me, but in consequence of its quantity and massive weight.

If, then, cold or heat be serviceable in bodily ailments like frost-bites or burns, they are so solely on account of their degree of temperature, just as they only inflict injury on the healthy body by their extreme degrees of temperature.

Thus we find in these examples of successful domestic practice, that it is not the prolonged application of the degree of cold in which the limb was frozen that restores it *isopathically* (it would thereby be rendered quite lifeless and dead), but a degree of cold that only approximates to that (*homœopathy*), and which gradually rises to a comfortable temperature, as frozen sour crout laid upon the frost-bitten hand in the temperature of the room soon melts, gradually growing warmer from 32° or 33° (Fahr.) to the temperature of the room, supposing that to be only 55°, and thus the limb is recovered by physical homœopathy. In like manner, a hand scalded with boiling water would not be cured *isopathically* by the application of boiling water, but only by a somewhat lower temperature, as, for example, by holding it in a vessel containing a fluid heated to 160°, which becomes every minute less hot, and finally descends to the temperature of the

heed the increase of pain that takes place at first, as he knows from experience that he can thereby in a very

---

room, whereupon the scalded part is restored by *homœopathy*. Water in the act of freezing cannot draw out the frost *isopathically* from potatoes and apples, but this is effected by water only near the freezing-point.

So, to give another example from physical action, the injury resulting from a blow on the forehead with a hard substance (a painful lump) is soon diminished in pain and swelling by pressing on the spot for a considerable time with the ball of the thumb, strongly at first, and then gradually less forcibly, homœopathically, but not by an equally hard blow with an equally hard body, which would increase the evil isopathically.

The examples of cures by isopathy given in the book alluded to —muscular contractions in human beings and spinal paralysis in a dog, which had been caused by a chill, being rapidly cured by cold bathing—these events are falsely explained by isopathy. What are called sufferings from a chill are only nominally connected with cold, and often arise, in the bodies of those predisposed to them, even from a draught of wind which was not at all cold. Moreover, the manifold effects of a cold bath on the living organism, in health and in disease, cannot be reduced to such a simple formula as to warrant the construction of a system of such pretentions! That serpents' bites, as is there stated, are most certainly cured by portions of the serpents, must remain a mere fable of a former age, until such an improbable assertion is authenticated by indubitable observations and experience, which it certainly never will be. That, in fine, the saliva of a mad dog given to a patient laboring under hydrophobia (in Russia), *is said* to have cured him—that "*is said*" would not seduce any conscientious physician to imitate such a hazardous experiment, or to construct a so-called isopathic system, so dangerous and so highly improbable in its extended application, as has been done (not by the modest author of the pamphlet entitled *The Isopathy of Contagions,* Leipzic: Kollmann, but) by its eccentric supporters, especially Dr. Gross (v. *Alg. hom. Ztg.,* ii, p. 72), who vaunts this isopathy (*æqualia*

short time, often in a few minutes, convert the burnt part into healthy painless skin.[33]

Other intelligent non-medical persons, as, for example, the manufacturers of lackered ware, apply to a part scalded with the hot varnish a substance that causes a similar *burning* sensation, such as strong heated *spirits of wine,*[34] or *oil of turpentine,*[35] and by that means cure

----

æqualibus) as the only proper therapeutic rule, and sees nothing in the *similia similibus* but an indifferent substitute for it; ungratefully enough, as he is entirely indebted to the *similia similibus* for all his fame and fortune.

[33] So also Fernelius (*Therap.*, lib. vi, cap. 20) considers that the best remedy for a burnt part is to bring it near the fire, whereby the pain is removed. John Hunter (*On the Blood, Inflammation,* etc., p. 218) mentions the great injury that results from treating burns with cold water, and gives a decided preference to approaching them to the fire, guided in this not by the traditional medical doctrines which (*contraria contrariis*) prescribe cooling things for inflammation, but by experience, which teaches that the application of a similar heat (*similia similibus*) is the most salutary.

[34] Sydenham (*Opera,* p. 271 [edit. Syd. Soc., p. 601]) says the *spirits of wine,* repeatedly applied, is preferable to all other remedies in burns. Benjamin Bell, too (*System of Surgery,* 3rd edit., 1789), acknowledges that experience shows that homœopathic remedies only are efficacious. He says: "One of the best applications to every burn of this kind is strong brandy or any other ardent spirit; it seems to induce a momentary additional pain (see below, § 157), but this soon subsides, and is succeeded by an agreeable soothing sensation. It proves most effectual when the parts can be kept immersed in it; but where this cannot be done, they should be kept constantly moist with pieces of old linen soaked in spirits." To this I may add that *warm, and indeed, very warm, alcohol is much more rapidly and much more certainly efficacious, for it is much more homœopathic than when not heated.* And all experience confirms this in a most astonishing manner.

[35] Edward Kentish, having to treat the workers in coal pits, who were so often dreadfully burnt by the explosion of fire-damp, ap-

themselves in the course of a few hours, whereas cooling salves, as they are well aware, would not effect a cure

---

plied heated oil of turpentine or alcohol, as the best remedy in the most extensive and severest burns (*Second Essay on Burns;* London, 1798). No treatment can be more homœopathic than this nor is any more efficacious.

The estimable and experienced Heister (*Institut. Chirurg.*, Tom. i, p. 33) confirms this from his own observation and extols the application of turpentine oil, of alcohol and of very hot poultices for this end, as hot as ever they can be borne.

But the amazing superiority of the application to burns of these remedies, which possess the power of exciting burning sensation and heat (and are consequently homœopathic), over palliative refrigerant remedies, is most incontestably shown by *pure* experimentation, in which the two opposite methods of treatment are employed for the sake of comparison, in burns of equal intensity in the same body.

Thus Benjamin Bell (in *Kühn's Phys. Med. Journ.*, Leipzic, 1801, Jun., p. 428), in the case of a lady who had scalded both arms, caused one to be covered with *oil of turpentine,* and made her plunge the other into *cold water.* In half an hour the first arm was *well,* but the other continued to be painful for six hours longer; when it was withdrawn one instant from the water she experienced much greater pain in it, *and it required a much longer time than the first for its cure.*

John Anderson (*Kentish,* op. cit., p. 43) treated in a similar manner a lady who had scalded herself with boiling grease. "The face which was very red and scalded and excessively painful was, a few minutes after the accident, covered with *oil of turpentine;* her arms she had, of her own accord, plunged into cold water, with which she desired to treat it for some hours. In the course of seven hours her face looked much better, and the pain was relieved. She had frequently renewed the cold water for the arm, but whenever she withdrew it she complained of much pain, and, in truth, the inflammation in it had *increased.* The following morning I found that she had had during the night great pain

in as many months, and cold water[36] would but make matters worse.

The old experienced reaper, although he may not be in the habit of drinking brandy, will not touch cold water (*contraria contrariis*) when he has worked himself into a violent feverish state in the heat of the sun—he knows the danger of such a proceeding—but he takes a small quantity of a *heating* liquor, a mouthful of brandy; experience, the teacher of truth, has convinced him of the great superiority and efficacy of this homœopathic procedure, whereby his heat and fatigue are speedily removed.[37]

There have occasionally been physicians who *vaguely surmised* that medicines cure analogous morbid states by

---

in the arm; the inflammation had extended above the elbow; several large blisters had risen, and thick eschars had formed on the arm and hand; a warm poultice was then applied. The face was completely free from pain, but emollient applications had to be used for the arm for a fortnight longer, before it was cured."

Who can fail to perceive in this instance the infinite superiority of the (homœopathic) *treatment by means of remedies of similar action, over the wretched treatment by opposites* (contraria contrariis) *of the antiquated ordinary school of medicine!*

[36] John Hunter (loc. cit.) is not singular in asserting the great injury done by treating burns with cold water. W. Fabricius of Hilden, also (*De Combustionibus libellus*, Basil, 1607, cap. 5, p. 11), alleges that cold applications in burns are highly injurious and productive of the most serious consequences; inflammation, suppuration and sometimes mortification are caused by them.

[37] Zimmerman (*Ueber die Erfahrung*, ii, p. 318) informs us that the inhabitants of hot countries act in the same manner, with the best results, and that, after being very much heated, they swallow a small quantity of some spirituous liquor.

the power they possess of producing analogous morbid symptoms.[88]

Thus the author of the book: περὶ τόπων κὰτ' ἀνθρώπον,[39] which is among the writings attributed to Hippocrates, has the following remarkable words: διὰ τὰ ὅμοια νοῦσος γίνεται, καί διὰ τὰ ὅμοια προσφερόμενα ἐκ νοσεύντων ὑγιαίνονται,—διὰ τὸ ἐμέειν ἔμετος παύεται.

Later physicians have also felt and expressed the truth of the homœopathic method of cure. Thus, for instance, Boulduc[40] perceived that the purgative property of rhubarb was the cause of its power to allay diarrhœa.

Detharding[41] guessed that the infusion of senna leaves relieved colic in adults by virtue of its analogous action in causing colic in healthy persons.

Bertholon[42] confesses that in diseases electricity diminishes and removes pain very similar to that which itself produces.

Thoury[43] testifies that positive electricity possesses the power of quickening the pulse, but when that is already morbidly accelerated it diminishes its frequency.

---

[88] I do not bring forward the following passages from authors who had a presentiment of homœopathy as proofs in support of this doctrine, which is firmly established by its own intrinsic merits, but in order to avoid the imputation of having suppressed these foreshadowings with the view of claiming for myself the priority of the idea.

[39] *Basil. Froben.*, 1538, p. 72.

[40] *Mémoirs de l' Académie Royale*, 1710.

[41] *Eph. Nat. Cur.*, cent. x, obs. 76.

[42] *Medicin. Electrisitat.*, ii, pp. 15 and 282.

[43] *Mémoir lu à l' Académie de Caen.*

Von Stoerk[44] makes the following suggestion: "If stramonium disorders the mind and produces mania in healthy persons, ought we not to try if in cases of insanity it cannot restore reason by producing a revolution in the ideas?"

But à Danish army physician, of the name of Stahl,[45] has expressed his conviction on this point in the most unequivocal terms. "The rule generally acted on in medicine," says he, "to treat by means of oppositely acting remedies (*contraria contrariis*), is quite false and the reverse of what ought to be; I am, on the contrary, convinced that diseases will yield to, and be cured by, remedies that produce a similar affection (*similia similibus*),—burns by exposure to the fire, frost-bitten limbs by the application of snow and the coldest water, inflammation and bruises by distilled spirits; and in like manner I have treated a tendency to acidity of the stomach by a very small dose of sulphuric acid with the most successful result, in cases where a number of absorbent remedies had been fruitlessly employed."

How near was the great truth sometimes of being apprehended! But it was dismissed with a mere passing thought, and thus the indispensable change of the antiquated medical treatment of disease, of the improper therapeutic system hitherto in vogue, into a real, true, and certain healing art, remained to be accomplished in our own times.

---

[44] *Libell. de Stram.*, p. 8.

[45] In Jo. Hammelii, *Commentatio de Arthritide tam tartarea, quam scorbutica, seu podagra et scorbuto*, Budingæ, 1738, viii, pp. 40-42.

ORGANON OF MEDICINE.

§ 1.

The physician's high and *only* mission is to restore the sick to health, to cure, as it is termed.[1]

§ 2.

The highest ideal of cure is rapid, gentle and permanent restoration of the health, or removal and annihilation of the disease in its whole extent, in the shortest, most reliable, and most harmless way, on easily comprehensible principles.

§ 3.

If the physician clearly perceives what is to be cured in diseases, that is to say, in every individual case of disease (*knowledge of disease, indication*), if he clearly

---

[1] His mission is not, however, to construct so-called systems, by interweaving empty speculations and hypotheses concerning the internal essential nature of the vital processes and the mode in which diseases originate in the invisible interior of the organism, (whereon so many physicians have hitherto ambitiously wasted their talents and their time); nor is it to attempt to give countless explanations regarding the phenomena in diseases and their proximate cause (which must ever remain concealed), wrapped in unintelligible words and an inflated abstract mode of expression,

perceives what is curative in medicines, that is to say, in each individual medicine (*knowledge of medicinal powers*), and if he knows how to adapt, according to clearly defined principles, what is curative in medicines to what he has discovered to be undoubtedly morbid in the patient, so that the recovery must ensue—to adapt it, as well in respect to the suitability of the medicine most appropriate according to its mode of action to the case before him (*choice of the remedy, the medicine indicated*), as also in respect to the exact mode of preparation and quantity of it required (*proper dose*), and the proper period for repeating the dose;—if, finally, he knows the obstacles to recovery in each case and is aware how to remove them, so that the restoration may be permanent, *then he understands how to treat judiciously and rationally, and he is a true practitioner of the healing art.*

§ 4.

He is likewise a preserver of health if he knows the things that derange health and cause disease, and how to remove them from persons in health.

---

which should sound very learned in order to astonish the ignorant—whilst sick humanity sighs in vain for aid. Of such learned reveries (to which the name of *theoretic medicine* is given, and for which special professorships are instituted) we have had quite enough, and it is now high time that all who call themselves physicians should at length cease to deceive suffering mankind with mere talk, and *begin* now, instead, for once to *act,* that is, really to help and to cure.

§ 5.

Useful to the physician in assisting him to cure are
the particulars of the most probable *exciting cause* of
the acute disease, as also the most significant points in
the whole history of the chronic disease, to enable him to
discover its *fundamental cause,* which is generally due to
a chronic miasm. In these investigations, the ascertainable physical constitution of the patient (especially when
the disease is chronic), his moral and intellectual character, his occupation, mode of living and habits, his social
and domestic relations, his age, sexual function, etc., are
to be taken into consideration.

§ 6.

The unprejudiced observer—well aware of the futility
of transcendental speculations which can receive no confirmation from experience—be his powers of penetration
ever so great, takes note of nothing in every individual
disease, except the changes in the health of the body and
of the mind (*morbid phenomena, accidents, symptoms*)
which can be perceived externally by means of the senses;
that is to say, he notices only the deviations from the
former healthy state of the now diseased individual,
which are felt by the patient himself, remarked by those
around him and observed by the physician. All these
perceptible signs represent the disease in its whole extent,
that is, together they form the true and only conceivable
portrait of the disease.[2]

---

[2] I know not, therefore, how it was possible for physicians at
the sick-bed to allow themselves to suppose that, without most

§ 7.

Now, as in a disease, from which no manifest exciting or maintaining cause (*causa occasionalis*) has to be removed,[a] we can perceive nothing but the morbid symptoms, it must (regard being had to the possibility of a miasm, and attention paid to the accessory circumstances, §5) be the symptoms alone by which the disease

---

carefully attending to the symptoms and being guided by them in the treatment, they ought to seek and could discover, only in the hidden and unknown interior, what there was to be cured in the disease, arrogantly and ludicrously pretending that they could, without paying much attention to the symptoms, discover the alteration that had occurred in the invisible interior, and set it to rights with (unknown!) medicines, and that such a procedure as this could alone be called radical and rational treatment.

Is not, then, that which is cognizable by the senses in diseases through the phenomena it displays, the disease itself in the eyes of the physician, since he never can see the spiritual being that produces the disease, the vital force? nor is it necessary that he should see it, but only that he should ascertain its morbid actions, in order that he may thereby be enabled to cure the disease. What else will the old school search for in the hidden interior of the organism, as a *prima causa morbi*, whilst they reject as an object of cure and contemptuously despise the sensible and manifest representation of the disease, the symptoms, that so plainly address themselves to us? What else do they wish to cure in diseases, but these?

[a] It is not necessary to say that every intelligent physician would first remove this where it exists; the indisposition thereupon generally ceases spontaneously. He will remove from the room strong-smelling flowers, which have a tendency to cause syncope and hysterical sufferings; extract from the cornea the foreign body that excites inflammation of the eye; loosen the over-tight band-

demands and points to the remedy suited to relieve it—and, moreover, the totality of these its symptoms, *of this outwardly reflected picture of the internal essence of the disease, that is, of the affection of the vital force*, must be the principal, or the sole means, whereby the disease can make known what remedy it requires—the only thing that can determine the choice of the most appropriate remedy—and thus, in a word, the totality[4] of the symptoms must be the principal, indeed the only, thing the physician has to take note of in every case of disease and to *remove* by means of his art, in order that the disease shall be cured and transformed into health.

---

age on a wounded limb that threatens to cause mortification, and apply a more suitable one; lay bare and put a ligature on the wounded artery that produces fainting; endeavor to promote the expulsion by vomiting of belladonna berries, etc., that may have been swallowed; extract foreign substances that may have got into the orifices of the body (the nose, gullet, ears, urethra, rectum, vagina); crush the vesical calculus; open the imperforate anus of the new-born infant, etc.

[4] In all times, the old school physicians, not knowing how else to give relief, have sought to combat and if possible to suppress by medicines, here and there, a *single* symptom from among a number in diseases—a *one-sided* procedure, which, under the name of *symptomatic treatment*, has justly excited universal contempt, because by it, not only was nothing gained, but much harm was inflicted. A single one of the symptoms present is no more the disease itself than a single foot is the man himself. This procedure was so much the more reprehensible, that such a single symptom was only treated by an antagonistic remedy (therefore only in an enantiopathic and palliative manner), whereby, after a slight alleviation, it was subsequently only rendered all the worse.

§ 8.

It is not conceivable, nor can it be proved by any experience in the world, that, after removal of all the symptoms of the disease and of the entire collection of the perceptible phenomena, there should or could remain anything else besides health, or that the morbid alteration in the interior could remain uneradicated.[5]

§ 9.

In the healthy condition of man, the spiritual vital force (autocracy), the dynamis that animates the material body (organism), rules with unbounded sway, and

---

[5] When a patient has been cured of his disease by a true physician, in such a manner that no trace of the disease, no morbid symptom, remains, and all the signs of health have permanently returned, how can anyone, without offering an insult to common sense, affirm in such an individual the whole bodily disease still remains in the interior? And yet the chief of the old school, Hufeland, asserts this in the following words: "Homœopathy can remove the symptoms, but the disease remains." (Vide *Homöopathie*, p. 27, I, 19.) This he maintains partly from mortification at the progress made by homœopathy to the benefit of mankind, partly because he still holds thoroughly material notions respecting disease, which he is still unable to regard as a state of being of the organism wherein it is dynamically altered by the morbidly deranged vital force, as an altered state of health, but he views the disease as *a something material*, which, after the cure is completed, may still remain lurking in some corner in the interior of the body, in order, some day during the most vigorous health, to burst forth at its pleasure with its material presence! So dreadful is still the blindness of the old pathology! No wonder

retains all the parts of the organism in admirable, harmonious, vital operation, as regards both sensations and functions, so that our indwelling, reason-gifted mind can freely employ this living, healthy instrument for the higher purposes of our existence.

§ 10.

The material organism, without the vital force, is capable of no sensation, no function, no self preservation;[6] it derives all sensation and performs all the functions of life solely by means of the immaterial being (the vital principle) which animates the material organism in health and in disease.

§ 11.

When a person falls ill, it is only this spiritual, self-acting (automatic) vital force, everywhere present in his organism, that is primarily deranged by the dynamic* influence upon it of a morbific agent inimical to life; it is only the vital principle, deranged to such an abnormal state, that can furnish the organism with its disagreeable sensations, and incline it to the irregular processes which

---

that it could only produce a system of therapeutics which is solely occupied with scouring out the poor patient.

[6] It is dead, and now only subject to the power of the external physical world; it decays, and is again resolved into its chemical constituents.

*Materia peccans!

we call disease; for, as a power invisible in itself, and only cognizable by its effects on the organism, its morbid derangement only makes itself known by the manifestation of disease in the sensations and functions of those parts of the organism exposed to the senses of the observer and physician, that is, by *morbid symptoms,* and in no other way can it make itself known.[7]

§ 12.

It is the morbidly affected vital energy alone that pro-

---

[7] What is dynamic influence,—dynamic power? Our earth, by virtue of a hidden invisible energy, carries the moon around her in twenty-eight days and several hours, and the moon alternately, in definite fixed hours (deducting certain differences which occur with the full and the new moon) raises our northern seas to flood tide and again correspondingly lowers them to ebb. Apparently this takes place not through material agencies, not through mechanical contrivances, as are used for products of human labor; and so we see numerous other events about us as results of the action of one substance on another substance without being able to recognize a sensible connection between cause and effect. Only the cultured, practised in comparison and deduction, can form for himself a kind of supra-sensual idea sufficient to keep all that is material or mechanical in his thoughts from such concepts. He calls such effects dynamic, virtual, that is, such as result from absolute, specific, pure energy and action of the one substance upon the other substance.

For instance, the dynamic effect of the sick-making influences upon healthy man, as well as the dynamic energy of the medicines upon the principle of life in the restoration of health is nothing else than infection and so not in any way material, not in any way mechanical. Just as the energy of a magnet attracting a piece of iron or steel is not material, not mechanical. One sees that the piece of iron is attracted by one pole of the magnet, but *how* it is done is not seen. This invisible energy of the magnet does not require mechanical (material) auxiliary means, hook or lever, to attract the iron. The magnet draws to itself and this acts upon the piece of iron or upon a steel needle by means of a purely immaterial, invisible, conceptual, inherent energy, that is, dynamically, and communicates to the steel needle the magnetic energy equally invisibly (dynamically). The steel needle becomes itself magnetic, even at a distance when the magnet does not touch it, and magnetises other steel needles with the same magnetic property (dynamically) with which it had been endowed previously by the magnetic rod, just as a child with small-pox or measles communicates to a near, untouched healthy child in an invisible manner (dynamically) the small-pox or measles, that is, infects it at a distance without anything material from the infective child going or capable of going to the one to be infected. A purely specific, conceptual influence communicated to the near child small-pox or measles in the same way as the magnet communicated to the near needle the magnetic property.

In a similar way, the effect of medicines upon living man is to be judged. Substances, which are used as medicines, are medicines only in so far as they possess each its own specific energy to alter the well-being of man through dynamic, conceptual influence, by means of the living sensory fibre, upon the conceptual, controlling principle of life. The medicinal property of those material substances which we call medicines proper, relates only to their energy to call out alterations in the well-being of animal life. Only upon this conceptual principle of life, depends their medicinal health-altering, conceptual (dynamic) influence. Just as the nearness of a magnetic pole can communicate only magnetic energy to the steel (namely, by a kind of infection) but cannot communicate other properties (for instance, more hardness or ductility, etc.). And thus every special medicinal substance alters through a kind of infection, that well-being of man in a peculiar manner exclusively its own and not in a manner peculiar to another medicine, as certainly as the nearness of the child ill with small-pox will communicate to a healthy child only small-pox and not measles. These medicines act upon our well-being wholly without communication of material parts of the medicinal substances, thus dynamically, as if through infection. Far more healing energy is expressed in a case in point by the smallest dose of the best dynamized medicines, in which there can be, according to calculation, only so little of material substance that its minuteness cannot be thought and conceived by the best arithmetical mind, than by large doses of the same medicine in substance. That smallest dose can therefore contain almost entirely only the pure, freely-developed, conceptual medicinal energy, and bring about only dynamically such great effects as can never be reached by the crude medicinal substance itself taken in large doses.

It is not in the corporeal atoms of these highly dynamized medicines, nor their physical or mathematical surfaces (with which the higher energies of the dynamized medicines are being interpreted but vainly as still sufficiently material) that the medicinal energy is found. More likely, there lies invisible in the moistened globule or in its solution, an unveiled, liberated, specific, medicinal force contained in the medicinal substance which acts dynamically by contact with the living animal fibre upon the whole organism (without communicating to it anything material however highly attenuated) and acts more strongly the more free and more immaterial the energy has become through the dynamization.

Is it then so utterly impossible for our age celebrated for its wealth in clear thinkers to think of dynamic energy as something non-corporeal, since we see daily phenomena which cannot be explained in any other manner? If one looks upon something nauseous and becomes inclined to vomit, did a material emetic come into his stomach which compels him to this anti-peristaltic movement? Was it not solely the dynamic effect of the nauseating aspect upon his imagination? And if one raises his arm, does it occur through a material visible instrument? a lever? Is it not solely the conceptual dynamic energy of his will which raises it?

duces diseases,[8] so that the morbid phenomena perceptible to our senses express at the same time all the internal change, that is to say, the whole morbid derangement of the internal dynamis; in a word, they reveal the whole disease; also, the disappearance under treatment of all the morbid phenomena and of all the morbid alterations that differ from the healthy vital operations, certainly affects and necessarily implies the restoration of the integrity of the vital force and, therefore, the recovered health of the whole organism.

§ 13.

Therefore disease (that does not come within the province of manual surgery) considered, as it is by the allopathists, as a thing separate from the living whole, from the organism and its animating vital force, and hidden in the interior, be it of ever so subtle a character, is an absurdity, that could only be imagined by minds of a materialistic stamp, and has for thousands of years given to the prevailing system of medicine all those pernicious impulses that have made it a truly mischievous [non-healing] art.

---

[8] *How* the vital force causes the organism to display morbid phenomena, that is, *how* it produces disease, it would be of no practical utility to the physician to know, and will forever remain concealed from him; only what it is necessary for him to know of the disease and what is fully sufficient for enabling him to cure it, has the Lord of life revealed to his senses.

§ 14.

There is, in the interior of man, nothing morbid that is curable and no visible morbid alteration that is curable which does not make itself known to the accurately observing physician by means of morbid signs and symptoms—an arrangement in perfect conformity with the infinite goodness of the all-wise Preserver of human life.

§ 15.

The affection of the morbidly deranged, spirit-like dynamis (vital force) that animates our body in the invisible interior, and the totality of the outwardly cognizable symptoms produced by it in the organism and representing the existing malady, constitute a whole; they are one and the same. The organism is indeed the material instrument of the life, but it is not conceivable without the animation imparted to it by the instinctively perceiving and regulating dynamis, just as the vital force is not conceivable without the organism, consequently the two together constitute a unity, although in thought our mind separates this unity into two distinct conceptions for the sake of easy comprehension.

§ 16.

Our vital force, as a spirit-like dynamis, cannot be attacked and affected by injurious influences on the healthy organism caused by the external inimical forces that disturb the harmonious play of life, otherwise than in a spirit-like (dynamic) way, and in like manner, all such morbid derangements (diseases) cannot be removed from it by the physician in any other way than by the spirit-like (dynamic⁹ virtual) alternative powers of the serviceable medicines acting upon our spirit-like vital force, which perceives them through the medium of the sentient faculty of the nerves everywhere present in the organism, so that it is only by their dynamic action on the vital force that remedies are able to re-establish and do actually re-establish health and vital harmony, after the changes in the health of the patient cognizable by our senses (the totality of the symptoms) have revealed the disease to the carefully observing and investigating physician as fully as was requisite in order to enable him to cure it.

§ 17.

Now, as in the cure effected by the removal of the whole of the perceptible signs and symptoms of the disease the internal alternation of the vital principle to which the disease is due—consequently the whole of the disease —is at the same time removed,[10] it follows that the

---

⁹ Most severe disease may be produced by sufficient disturbance of the vital force through the imagination and also cured by the same means.

¹⁰ A warning dream, a superstitious fancy, or a solemn prediction that death would occur at a certain day or at a certain hour, has not unfrequently produced all the signs of commencing and increasing disease, of approaching death and death itself at the hour announced, which could not happen without the simultaneous production of the inward change (corresponding to the state

physician has only to remove the whole of the symptoms in order, at the same time, to abrogate and annihilate the internal change, that is to say, the morbid derangement of the vital force—consequently the totality of the disease, the *disease itself.*[11] But when the disease is annihilated, health is restored, and this is the highest, the sole aim of the physician who knows the true object of his mission, which consists not in learned-sounding prating, but in giving aid to the sick.

§ 18.

From this indubitable truth, that besides the totality of the symptoms, with consideration of the accompanying

---

observed externally); and hence in such cases all the morbid signs indicative of approaching death have frequently been dissipated by an identical cause, by some cunning deception or persuasion to a belief in the contrary, and health suddenly restored, which could not have happened without the removal, by means of this moral remedy, of the internal and external morbid change that threatened death.

[11] It is only thus that God, the Preserver of mankind, could reveal His wisdom and goodness in reference to the cure of the diseases to which man is liable here below, by showing to the physician what he had to remove in diseases in order to annihilate them and thus re-establish health. But what would we think of His wisdom and goodness if He had shrouded in mysterious obscurity that which was to be cured in diseases (as is asserted by the dominant school of medicine, which affects to possess a supernatural insight into the inner nature of things), and shut it up in the hidden interior, and thus rendered it impossible for man to know the malady accurately, consequently impossible for him to cure it?

modalities (§ 5) nothing can by any means be discovered in diseases wherewith they could express their
need of aid, it follows undeniably that the sum of all the
symptoms and conditions in each individual case of disease must be the *sole indication*, the sole guide to direct
us in the choice of a remedy.

§ 19.

Now, as *diseases* are nothing more than *alterations in
the state of health of the healthy individual* which express
themselves by morbid signs, and the *cure* is also only
possible by a *change to the healthy condition of the state
of health of the diseased individual,* it is very evident
that *medicines* could never cure diseases if they did not
possess the power of altering man's state of health which
depends on sensations and functions; indeed, that their
curative power must be owing *solely* to this power they
possess of altering man's state of health.

§ 20.

This spirit-like power to alter man's state of health
which lies hidden in the inner nature of medicines can
in itself never be discovered by us by a mere effort of
reason; it is only by experience of the phenomena it
displays when acting on the state of health of man that
we can become clearly cognizant of it.

§ 21.

Now, as it is undeniable that the curative principle in
medicines is not in itself perceptible, and as in pure ex-

periments with medicines conducted by the most accurate observers, nothing can be observed that can constitute them medicines or remedies except that power of causing distinct alterations in the state of health of the human body, and particularly in that of the *healthy individual,* and of exciting in him various definite morbid symptoms; so it follows that when medicines act as remedies, they can only bring their curative property into play by means of this their power of altering man's state of health by the production of peculiar symptoms; and that, therefore, we have only to rely on the morbid phenomena which the medicines produce in the healthy body as the sole possible revelation of their in-dwelling curative power, in order to learn what disease-producing power, and at the same time what disease-curing power, each individual medicine possesses.

§ 22.

But as nothing is to be observed in diseases that must be removed in order to change them into health besides the totality of their signs and symptoms, and likewise medicines can show nothing curative besides their tendency to produce morbid symptoms in healthy persons and to remove them in diseased persons; it follows, on the one hand, that medicines only become remedies and capable of annihilating diseases, because the medicinal substance, by exciting certain effects and symptoms, that is to say, by producing a certain artificial morbid state, removes and abrogates the symptoms already present, to wit, the natural morbid state we wish to cure. On the

other hand, it follows that, for the totality of the symptoms of the disease to be cured, that medicine must be
sought which (according as experience shall prove
whether the morbid symptoms are most readily, certainly,
and permanently removed and changed into health by
similar or *opposite* medicinal symptoms[12]) proved to have

---

[12] The other possible mode of employing medicines for diseases besides these two is the *allopathic method,* in which medicines are given, whose symptoms have no direct pathological relation to the morbid state, neither similar nor opposite, but quite
heterogeneous to the symptoms of the disease. This procedure
plays, as I have shown elsewhere, an irresponsible murderous
game with the life of the patient by means of dangerous, violent medicines, whose action is unknown and which are chosen
on mere conjectures and given in large and frequent doses.
Again, by means of painful operations, intended to lead the disease to other regions and taking the strength and vital juices of
the patient, through evacuations above and below, sweat or salivation, but especially through squandering the irreplaceable blood,
as is done by the reigning routine practice, used blindly and re-
lentlessly, usually with the pretext that the physician should imitate and further the sick nature in its efforts to help itself, without considering how irrational it is, to imitate and further these
very imperfect, mostly inappropriate efforts of the instinctive
unintelligent vital energy which is implanted in our organism, so
long as it is healthy to carry on life in harmonious development, but not to heal itself in disease. For, were it possessed of
such a model ability, it would never have allowed the organism
to get sick. When made ill by noxious agents, our life principle cannot do anything else than express its depression caused
by disturbance of the regularity of its life, by symptoms, by
means of which the intelligent physician is asked for aid. If
this is not given, it strives to save by increasing the ailment,
especially through violent evacuations, no matter what this en-

the greatest tendency to produce similar or opposite symptoms.

§ 23.

All pure experience, however, and all accurate research convince us that persistent symptoms of disease are far from being removed and annihilated by *opposite* symptoms of medicines (as in the *antipathic, enantiopathic* or *palliative* method), that, on the contrary, after transient, apparent alleviation, they break forth again, only with increased intensity, and become manifestly aggravated (see § 58-62 and 69).

§ 24.

There remains, therefore, no other mode of employing medicines in diseases that promises to be of service besides the homœopathic, by means of which we seek, for the totality of the symptoms of the case of disease, a medicine which among all medicines (whose pathogenetic effects are known from having been tested in healthy individuals) has the power and the tendency to produce an artificial morbid state most similar to that of the case of disease in question.

---

tails, often with the largest sacrifices or destruction of life itself.

For purposes of cure, the morbidly depressed vital energy possesses so little ability worthy of imitation since all changes and symptoms produced by it in the organism are the disease itself. What intelligent physician would want to imitate it with the intention to heal if he did not thereby sacrifice his patient?

§ 25.

Now, however, in all careful trials, pure experience,[13] the sole and infallible oracle of the healing art, teaches us that actually that medicine which, in its action on the healthy human body, has demonstrated its power of producing the greatest number of symptoms *similar* to those observable in the case of disease under treatment, does also, in doses of suitable potency and attenuation, rapidly, radically and permanently remove the totality of the symptoms of this morbid state, that is to say (§ 6-16), the whole disease present, and change it into health; and that all medicines cure, without exception, those diseases whose symptoms most nearly resemble their own, and leave none of them uncured.

---

[13] I do not mean that sort of experience of which the ordinary practitioners of the old school boast, after they have for years worked away with a lot of complex prescriptions on a number of diseases which they never carefully investigated, but which, faithful to the tenets of their school, they considered as already described in works of systematic pathology, and dreamed that they could detect in them some imaginary morbific matter, or ascribed to them some other hypothetical internal abnormality. They always saw something in them, but knew not what it was they saw, and they got results, from the complex forces acting on an unknown object, that no human being but only a God could have unravelled—results from which nothing can be learned, no experience gained. Fifty years' experience of this sort is like fifty years of looking into a kaleidoscope filled with unknown colored objects, and perpetually turning round; thousands of ever-changing figures and no accounting for them!

§ 26.

This depends on the following homœopathic law of nature which was sometimes, indeed, vaguely surmised but not hitherto fully recognized, and to which is due every real cure that has ever taken place:

A weaker dynamic affection is permanently extinguished in the living organism by a stronger one, if the latter (whilst differing in kind) is very similar to the former in its manifestations.[14]

---

[14] Thus are cured both physical affections and moral maladies. How is it that in the early dawn the brilliant Jupiter vanishes from the gaze of the beholder? By a stronger very similar power acting on his optic nerve, the brightness of approaching day!—In situations replete with fœtid odors, wherewith is it usual to soothe effectually the offended olfactory nerves? With snuff, that affects the sense of smell in a similar but stronger manner! No music, no sugared cake, which act on the nerves of other senses, can cure this olfactory disgust. How does the soldier cunningly stifle the piteous cries of him who runs the gauntlet from the ears of the compassionate bystanders? By the shrill notes of the fife commingled with the roll of the noisy drum! And the distant roar of the enemy's cannon that inspires his army with fear? By the loud boom of the big drum! For neither the one nor the other would the distribution of a brilliant piece of uniform nor a reprimand to the regiment suffice.—In like manner, mourning and sorrow will be effaced from the mind by the account of another and still greater cause for sorrow happening to another, even though it be a mere fiction. The injurious consequences of too great joy will be removed by drinking coffee, which produces an excessively joyous state of mind. Nations like the Germans, who have for centuries been gradually sinking deeper and deeper in soulless apathy and degrading serfdom, must first be trodden still deeper

§ 27.

The curative power of medicines, therefore, depends on their symptoms, similar to the disease but superior to it in strength (§ 12-26), so that each individual case of disease is most surely, radically, rapidly and permanently annihilated and removed only by a medicine capable of producing (in the human system) in the most similar and complete manner the totality of its symptoms, which at the same time are stronger than the disease.

§ 28.

As this natural law of cure manifests itself in every pure experiment and every true observation in the world, the fact is consequently established; it matters little what may be the scientific explanation of *how it takes place;* and I do not attach much importance to the attempts made to explain it. But the following view seems to commend itself as the most probable one, as it is founded on premises derived from experience.

§ 29.

As every disease (not entirely surgical) consists only in a special, morbid, dynamic alteration of our vital energy (of the principle of life) manifested in sensation

in the dust by the Western Conqueror, until their situation became intolerable; their mean opinion of themselves was thereby overstrained and removed; they again became alive to their dignity as men, and then, for the first time, they raised their heads as Germans,

and motion, so in every homœopathic cure this principle of life dynamically altered by natural disease is seized through the administration of a medicinal potency selected exactly according to symptom-similarity by a somewhat stronger, similar artificial disease-manifestation. By this the feeling of the natural (weaker) dynamic disease-manifestation ceases and disappears. This disease-manifestation no longer exists for the principle of life which is now occupied and governed merely by the stronger, artificial disease-manifestation. This artificial disease-manifestation has soon spent its force and leaves the patient free from disease, cured. The dynamis, thus freed, can now continue to carry life on in health. This most highly probable process rests upon the following propositions.

§ 30.

The human body appears to admit of being much more powerfully affected in its health by medicines (partly because we have the regulation of the dose in our own power) than by natural morbid stimuli—for natural diseases are cured and overcome by suitable medicines.[15]

---

[15] The short duration of the action of the artificial morbific forces, which we term medicines, makes it possible that, although they are stronger than the natural diseases, they can yet be much more easily overcome by the vital force than can the weaker natural diseases, which, solely in consequence of the longer, generally lifelong, duration of their action (psora, syphilis, sycosis), can never be vanquished and extinguished by it

§ 31.

The inimical forces, partly psychical, partly physical, to which our terrestrial existence is exposed, which are termed morbific noxious agents, do not possess the power of morbidly deranging the health of man unconditionally;[16] but we are made ill by them only when our organism is sufficiently disposed and susceptible to the attack of the morbific cause that may be present, and to be altered in its health, deranged and made to undergo abnormal sensations and functions—hence they do not produce disease in every one nor at all times.

§ 32.

But it is quite otherwise with the artificial morbific agents which we term medicines. Every real medicine, namely, acts at *all* times, under *all* circumstances, on *every* living human being, and produces in him its peculiar symptoms (distinctly perceptible, if the dose be large

---

alone, until the physician affects the vital force in a stronger manner by an agent that produces a disease very similar, but stronger, to wit a homœopathic medicine. The cures of diseases of many years' duration (§ 46), by the occurrence of smallpox and measles (both of which run a course of only a few weeks), are processes of a similar character.

[16] When I call disease a *derangement* of man's state of health, I am far from wishing thereby to give a *hyperphysical* explanation of the internal nature of diseases generally, or of any case of disease in particular. It is only intended by this expression to intimate, what it can be proved diseases are *not* and *cannot be,* that they are not mechanical or chemical alterations of the

enough), so that evidently every living human organism is liable to be affected, and, as it were, inoculated with the medicinal disease at all times, and absolutely (*unconditionally*), which, as before said, is by no means the case with the natural diseases.

§ 33.

In accordance with this fact, it is undeniably shown by all experience[17] that the living human organism is much more disposed and has a greater liability to be acted on, and to have its health deranged by medicinal powers, than by morbific noxious agents and infectious miasms, or, in other words, *that the morbific noxious agents possess a power of morbidly deranging man's health that is subordinate and conditional, often very conditional; whilst medicinal agents have an absolute unconditional power, greatly superior to the former.*

---

material substance of the body, and not dependent on a material morbific substance, but that they are merely spirit-like (conceptual) dynamic derangements of the life.

[17] A striking fact in corroboration of this is, that whilst previously to the year 1801, when the smooth scarlatina of Sydenham still occasionally prevailed epidemically among children, it attacked without exception all children who had escaped it in a former epidemic; in a similar epidemic which I witnessed in Königslutter, on the contrary, *all* the children who took in time a very small dose of belladonna remained unaffected by this highly infectious infantile disease. If medicines can protect from a disease that is raging around, they must possess a vastly superior power of affecting our vital force.

§ 34.

The greater strength of the artificial diseases producible by medicines is, however, not the sole cause of their power to cure natural diseases. In order that they may effect a cure, it is before all things requisite that they should be capable of producing in the human body *an artificial disease as similar as possible* to the disease to be cured, which, with somewhat increased power, transforms to a very similar morbid state the instinctive life principle, which in itself is incapable of any reflection or act of memory. It not only obscures, but extinguishes and thereby annihilates the derangement caused by the natural disease. This is so true, that no previously existing disease can be cured, even by Nature herself, by the accession of a new *dissimilar* disease, be it ever so strong, and just as little can it be cured by medical treatment with drugs which are incapable of producing a *similar* morbid condition in the healthy body.

§ 35.

In order to illustrate this, we shall consider in three different cases, as well what happens in nature when two dissimilar natural diseases meet together in one person, as also the result of the ordinary medical treatment of diseases with unsuitable allopathic drugs, which are incapable of producing an artificial morbid condition similar to the disease to be cured, whereby it will appear that even Nature herself is unable to remove a dissimilar disease already present by one that is unhomœopathic, even though it be stronger, and just as little is the un-homœopathic employment of even the strongest medicines ever capable of curing any disease whatsoever.

§ 36.

I. If the two *dissimilar* diseases meeting together in the human being be of equal strength, or still more if the *older one be the stronger,* the new disease will be repelled by the old one from the body and not allowed to affect it. A patient suffering from a severe chronic disease will not be infected by a moderate autumnal dysentery or other epidemic disease. The plague of the Levant, according to Larry,[18] does not break out where scurvy is prevalent, and persons suffering from eczema are not infected by it. Rachitis, Jenner alleges, prevents vaccination from taking effect. Those suffering from pulmonary consumption are not liable to be attacked by epidemic fevers of a not very violent character, according to Von Hildenbrand.

§ 37.

So, also, *under ordinary medical treatment,* an old chronic disease remains uncured and unaltered if it is treated according to the common *allopathic* method, that is to say, with medicines that are incapable of producing in healthy individuals a state of health similar to the

---

[18] "Mémoires et Observations," in the *Description de l' Egypte,* tom. i.

disease, even though the treatment should last for years and is not of too violent character.[19] This is daily witnessed in practice, it is therefore unnecessary to give any illustrative examples.

§ 38.

II. Or *the new dissimilar disease is the stronger.* In this case the disease under which the patient originally labored, being the weaker, will be kept back and suspended by the accession of the stronger one, until the latter shall have run its course or been cured, and then the old one reappears *uncured.* Two children affected with a kind of epilepsy remained free from epileptic attacks after infection with ringworm (*tinea*); but as soon as the eruption on the head was gone the epilepsy returned just as before, as Tulpius[20] observed. The itch, as Schöpf[21] saw, disappeared on the occurrence of the scurvy, but after the cure of the latter it again broke out. So also the pulmonary phthisis remained stationary when the patient was attacked by a violent typhus, but went on again after the latter had run its course.[22] If mania occur in a consumptive patient, the

---

[19] But if treated with violent allopathic remedies, other diseases will be formed in its place which are more difficult and dangerous to life.

[20] *Obs.,* lib. i, obs. 8.

[21] In *Hufeland's Journal,* xv, 2.

[22] Chevalier, in Hufeland's *Neuesten Annalen der französichen Heilkunde,* ii, p. 192.

phthisis with all its symptoms is removed by the former; but if that go off, the phthisis returns immediately and proves fatal.[23] When measles and smallpox are prevalent at the same time, and both attack the same child, the measles that had already broken out is generally checked by the smallpox that came somewhat later; nor does the measles resume its course until after the cure of the smallpox; but it not infrequently happens that the inoculated smallpox is suspended for four days by the supervention of the measles, as observed by Manget,[24] after the desquamation of which the smallpox completes its course. Even when the inoculation of the smallpox had taken effect for six days, and the measles then broke out, the inflammation of the inoculation remained stationary and the smallpox did not ensue until the measles had completed its regular course of seven days.[25] In an epidemic of measles, that disease attacked many individuals on the fourth or fifth day after the inoculation of smallpox and prevented the development of the smallpox until it had completed its own course, whereupon the smallpox appeared and proceeded regularly to its termination.[26] The true, smooth, erysipelatous-looking scarlatina of Sydenham,[27] with sore throat,

---

[23] Mania phthisi superveniens eam cum omnibus suis phænomenis auffert, verum mox redit phthisis et occidit, abeunte mania. Reil *Memorab.*, fasc. iii, v, p. 171.

[24] In the *Edinb. Med. Comment.*, pt. i, 1.

[25] John Hunter. *On the Venereal Disease*, p. 5.

[26] Rainey, in the *Edinb. Med. Comment.*, iii, p. 480.

[27] Very accurately described by Withering and Plenciz, but differing greatly from the purpura (or Roodvonk), which is often

was checked on the fourth day by the eruption of cow-pox, which ran its regular course, and not till it was ended did the scarlatina again establish itself; but on another occasion, as both diseases seem to be of equal strength, the cow-pox was suspended on the eighth day by the supervention of the true, smooth scarlatina of Sydenham, and the red areola of the former disappeared until the scarlatina was gone, whereon the cow-pox immediately resumed its course, and went on to its regular termination.[28] The measles suspended the cow-pox; on the eighth day, when the cow-pox had nearly attained its climax, the measles broke out; the cow-pox now remained stationary, and did not resume and complete its course until the desquamation of the measles had taken place, so that on the sixteenth day it presented the appearance it otherwise would have shown on the tenth day, as Kortum observed.[29]

Even after the measles had broken out the cow-pox inoculation took effect, but did not run its course until the measles had disappeared, as Kortum likewise witnessed.[30]

I myself saw the mumps (*angina parotidea*) immediately disappear when the cow-pox inoculation had taken effect and had nearly attained its height; it was

---

erroneously denominated scarlet fever. It is only of late years that the two, which were originally very different diseases, have come to resemble each other in their symptoms.

[28] Jenner, in *Medicinische Annalen*, August, 1800, p. 747.

[29] In *Hufeland's Journal der praktischen Arzneikunde*, xx, 3, p. 50.

[30] *Loc. cit.*

not until the complete termination of the cow-pox and the disappearance of its red arcola that this febrile tumefaction of the parotid and submaxillary glands, that is caused by a peculiar miasm, reappeared and ran its regular course of seven days.

And thus it is with all dissimilar diseases; the stronger suspends the weaker (when they do not complicate one another, which is seldom the case with acute diseases), *but they never cure one another*.

§ 39.

Now the adherents of the ordinary school of medicine saw all this for so many centuries; they saw that Nature herself cannot cure any disease by the accession of another, be it ever so strong, if the new disease be *dissimilar* to that already present in the body. What shall we think of them, that they nevertheless went on treating chronic diseases with allopathic remedies, namely, with medicines and prescriptions capable of producing God knows what morbid state—almost invariably, however, one *dissimilar* to the disease to be cured? And even though physicians did not hitherto observe nature attentively, the miserable results of their treatment should have taught them that they were pursuing an inappropriate, a false path. Did they not perceive when they employed, as was their custom, an aggressive allopathic treatment in a chronic disease, that thereby they only created an artificial disease *dissimilar* to the original one, which, as long as it was kept up, merely held in abeyance, merely suppressed, merely suspended the original disease, which latter, however, always returned, and must return, as soon as the diminished strength of the patient no longer admitted of a continuance of the allopathic attacks on the life? Thus the itch exanthema certainly disappears very soon from the skin under the employment of violent purgatives, frequently repeated; but when the patient can no longer stand the factitious (*dissimilar*) disease of the bowels, and can take no more purgatives, then either the cutaneous eruption breaks out as before, or the internal psora displays itself in some bad symptom, and the patient, in addition to his undiminished original disease, has to endure the misery of a painful ruined digestion and impaired strength to boot. So, also, when the ordinary physicians keep up artificial ulcerations of the skin and issues on the exterior of the body, with the view of thereby eradicating a chronic disease, they can NEVER attain their object by so doing, they can NEVER cure them by that means, as such artificial cutaneous ulcers are quite alien and allopathic to the internal affection; but inasmuch as the irritation produced by several tissues is at least sometimes a stronger (*dissimilar*) disease than the indwelling malady, the latter is thereby sometimes silenced and suspended for a week or two. But it is *only suspended,* and that for a very short time, whilst the patient's powers are gradually worn out. Epilepsy, suppressed for many years by means of issues, invariably recurred, and in an aggravated form, when they were allowed to heal up, as Pechlin [31] and others testify. But purgatives for itch, and issues for epilepsy, cannot be more heterogeneous,

---

[31] *Obs. phys. med.,* lib. ii, obs. 30.

more dissimilar deranging agents—cannot be more allopathic, more exhausting modes of treatment—than are the customary prescriptions, composed of unknown ingredients, used in ordinary practice for the other nameless, innumerable forms of disease. These likewise do nothing but debilitate, and only suppress or suspend the malady for a short time without being able to cure it, and when used for a long time always add a new morbid state to the old disease.

§ 40.

III. Or *the new disease,* after having long acted on the organism, at length *joins the old one that is dissimilar to it,* and forms with it a *complex* disease, so that each of them occupies a particular locality in the organism, namely, the organs peculiarly adapted to it, and, as it were, only the place specially belonging to it, whilst it leaves the rest to the other disease that is dissimilar to it. Thus a syphilitic patient may become psoric, and *vice versa. As two diseases dissimilar to each other, they cannot remove, cannot cure one another.* At first the venereal symptoms are kept in abeyance and suspended when the psoric eruption begins to appear; in course of time, however (as the syphilis is at least as strong as the psora), the two join together,[32] that is,

---

[32] From careful experiments and cures of complex diseases of this kind, I am now firmly convinced that no real amalgamation of the two takes place, but that in such cases the one exists in the organism *besides* the other only, each in the part that is adapted for it, and their cure will be completely effected by a

each involves those parts of the organism only which are most adapted for it, and the patient is thereby rendered more diseased and more difficult to cure.

When two dissimilar acute infectious diseases meet, as, for example, smallpox and measles, the one usually suspends the other, as has been before observed; yet there have also been severe epidemics of this kind, where, in rare cases, two dissimilar acute diseases occurred simultaneously in one and the same body, and for a short time combined, as it were, with each other. During an epidemic, in which smallpox and measles were prevalent at the same time, among three hundred cases (in which these diseases avoided or suspended one another, and the measles attacked patients twenty days after the smallpox broke out, the smallpox, however, from seventeen to eighteen days after the appearance of the measles, so that the first disease had previously completed its regular course) there was yet one single case in which P. Russell [33] met with both these dissimilar diseases in one person at the same time. Rainey [34] witnessed the simultaneous occurrence of smallpox and measles in two girls. J. Maurice,[35] in his whole practice, only observed two such cases. Similar cases are to be

---

judicious alteration of the best mercurial preparation, with the remedies specific for the psora, each given in the most suitable dose and form.

[33] Vide *Transactions of a Society for the Improvement of Med. and Chir. Knowledge*, ii.

[34] In *Edinb. Med. Comment.*, iii, p. 480.

[35] In *Med. and Phys. Journ.*, 1805.

found in Ettmüller's [86] works, and in the writings of a few others.

Zencker [87] saw cow-pox run its regular course along with measles and along with purpura.

The cow-pox went on its course undisturbed during a mercurial treatment for syphilis, as Jenner saw.

§ 41.

Much more frequent than the natural diseases associating with and complicating one another in the same body are the morbid complications which the inappropriate medical treatment (the allopathic method) is apt to produce by the long-continued employment of unsuitable drugs. To the natural disease, which it is proposed to cure, there are then added, by the constant repetition of the unsuitable medicinal agent, the new, often very tedious, morbid conditions corresponding to the nature of this agent; these gradually coalesce with and complicate the chronic malady which is dissimilar to them (which they were unable to cure by similarity of action, that is, homœopathically), adding to the old disease a new, dissimilar, artificial malady of a chronic nature, and thus give the patient a double in place of a single disease, that is to say, render him much worse and more difficult to cure, often quite incurable. Many of the cases for which advice is asked in medical journals, as also the records of other cases in medical

---

[86] *Opera,* ii, p. i., cap. 10.
[87] In *Hufeland's Journal,* xvii.

writings, attest the truth of this. Of a similar character are the frequent cases in which the venereal chancrous disease, complicated especially with psora or with the dyscrasia of condylomatous gonorrhœa, is not cured by long-continued or frequently repeated treatment with large doses of unsuitable mercurial preparations, but assumes its place in the organism beside the chronic mercurial affection [88] that has been in the meantime gradually developed, and thus along with it often forms a° hideous monster of complicated disease (under the general name of masked venereal disease), which then, when not quite incurable, can only be transformed into health with the greatest difficulty.

§ 42.

Nature herself permits, as has been stated, in some cases, the simultaneous occurrence of two (indeed, of three) natural diseases in one and the same body. This complication, however, it must be remarked, happens only in the case of two *dissimilar* diseases, which according to the eternal laws of nature do not remove, do not annihilate and cannot cure one another, but, as it seems, both (or all three) remain, as it were, separate in the

---

[88] For mercury, besides the morbid symptoms which by virtue of similarity can cure the venereal disease homœopathically, has among its effects many others unlike those of syphilis, for instance, swelling and ulceration of bones, which, if it be employed in large doses, causes new maladies and commits great ravages in the body, especially when complicated with psora, as is so frequently the case.

organism, and each takes possession of the parts and systems peculiarly appropriate to it, which, on account of the want of resemblance of these maladies to each other, can very well happen without disparagement to the unity of life.

§ 43.

Totally different, however, is the result when *two similar* diseases meet together in the organism, that is to say, when to the disease already present a stronger similar one is added. In such cases we see how a cure can be effected by the operations of nature, and we get a lesson as to how man ought to cure.

§ 44.

Two *similar* diseases can neither (as is asserted of dissimilar diseases in I) *repel* one another, nor (as has been shown of dissimilar diseases in II) *suspend* one another, so that the old one shall return after the new one has run its course; and just as little can two *similar* diseases (as has been demonstrated in III respecting dissimilar affections) *exist beside each other* in the same organism, or together form a *double* complex disease.

§ 45.

No! two diseases, differing, it is true, in kind,* but very similar in their phenomena and effects and in the

---

*Vide, *supra,* § 26, note.

sufferings and symptoms they severally produce, invariably annihilate one another whenever they meet together in the organism; the stronger disease, namely, annihilates the weaker, and that for this simple reason, because the stronger morbific power when it invades the system, by reason of its similarity of action involves precisely the *same* parts of the organism that were previously affected by the weaker morbid irritation, which, consequently, can no longer act on these parts, but is extinguished;[39] or (in other words), the new similar but stronger morbific potency controls the feelings of the patient and hence the life principle on account of its peculiarity, can no longer feel the weaker similar which becomes extinguished—exists no longer—for it was never anything material, but a dynamic—spirit-like—(conceptual) affection. The life principle henceforth is affected only and this but temporarily by the new, similar but stronger morbific potency.

§ 46.

Many examples might be adduced of diseases which, in the course of nature, have been homœopathically cured by other diseases presenting similar symptoms, were it not necessary, as our object is to speak about something determinate and indubitable, to confine our attention solely to those (few) diseases which are invariably the

---

[39] Just as the image of a lamp's flame is rapidly overpowered and effaced from our retina by the stronger sunbeam impinging on the eye.

same, arise from a fixed miasm, and hence merit a distinct name.

Among these the smallpox, so dreaded on account of the great number of its serious symptoms, occupies a prominent position, and it has removed and cured a number of maladies with similar symptoms.

How frequently does smallpox produce violent ophthalmia, sometimes even causing blindness! And see! by its inoculation Dezoteux [40] cured a chronic ophthalmia permanently, and Leroy [41] another.

An amaurosis of two years' duration, consequent on suppressed scald-head, was perfectly cured by it, according to Klein.[42]

How often does smallpox cause deafness and dyspnœa! And both these chronic diseases it removed on reaching its acme, as J. Fr. Closs [43] observed.

Swelling of the testicle, even of a very severe character, is a frequent symptom of smallpox, and on this account it was enabled, as Klein [44] observed, to cure, by virtue of similarity, a large hard swelling of the left testicle, consequent on a bruise. And another observer [45] saw a similar swelling of the testicle cured by it.

Among the troublesome symptoms of smallpox is a dysenteric state of the bowels; and it subdued, as Fr.

<hr>

[40] *Traité de l'inoculation*, p. 189.
[41] *Heilkunde für Mütter*, p. 384.
[42] *Interpres clinicus*, p. 293.
[43] *Neue Heilart der Kinderpocken*, Ulm, 1769, p. 68; and *Specim.*, obs. No. 18.
[44] *Op. cit.*
[45] *Nov. Act. Nat. cur.*, vol. i, obs. 22.

Wendt [46] observed, a case of dysentery, as a similar morbific agent.

Smallpox coming on after vaccination, as well on account of its greater strength as its great similarity, at once removes entirely the cow-pox homœopathically, and does not permit it to come to maturity; but, on the other hand, the cow-pox when near maturity does, on account of its great similarity, homœopathically diminish very much the supervening smallpox and make it much milder, [47] as Mühry [48] and many others testify.

The inoculated *cow-pox*, whose lymph, besides the protective matter, contains the contagion of a general cutaneous eruption of another nature, consisting of usually small, dry (rarely large, pustular) pimples, resting on a small red areola, frequently conjoined with round red cutaneous spots and often accompanied by the most violent itching, which rash appears in not a few children several days *before*, more frequently, however, *after* the red areola of the cow-pock, and goes off in a few days, leaving behind small, red, hard spots on the skin;—the inoculated cow-pox, I say, after it has taken cures perfectly and permanently, in a homœopathic

---

[46] *Nachricht von dem Krankeninstitut zu Erlangen,* 1783.

[47] This seems to be the reason for this beneficial remarkable fact namely that since the general distribution of Jenner's Cow Pox vaccination, human smallpox never again appeared as epidemically or virulently as 40-50 years before when one city visited lost at least one-half and often three-quarters of its children by death of this miserable pestilence.

[48] Willan, *Ueber die Kuhpockenimpfung, aus dem Engl., mit Zusätzen G. P. Mühry,* Göttingen, 1808.

manner, by the similarity of this accessory miasm, analogous cutaneous eruptions of children, often of very long standing and of a very troublesome character, as a number of observers assert.[49]

The cow-pox, a peculiar symptom of which is to cause tumefaction of the arm,[50] cured, after it broke out, a *swollen* half-paralyzed arm.[51]

The fever accompanying cow-pox, which occurs at the time of the production of the red areola, cured homœopathically intermittent fever in two individuals, as the younger Hardege[52] reports, confirming what J. Hunter[53] had already observed, that two fevers (similar diseases) cannot co-exist in the same body.

The *measles* bears a strong resemblance in the character of its fever and cough to the whooping-cough, and hence it was that Bosquillon[54] noticed, in an epidemic where both these affections prevailed, that many children who then took measles remained free from whooping-cough. They would all have been protected from, and rendered incapable of being infected by, the whooping-cough in that and all subsequent epidemics, by the measles, if the

---

[49] Especially Clavier, Hurel and Desmormeaux, in the *Bulletin des sciences médicales, publié par les membres du comité central de la Soc. de Médecine du Departement de l' Eure,* 1808; also in the *Journal de médicine continué,* vol. xv, p. 206.

[50] Balhorn, in *Hufeland's Journal,* 10, ii.

[51] Stevenson, in Duncan's *Annals of Medicine,* lustr. 2, vol. i, pt. 2, No. 9.

[52] In *Hufeland's Journal,* xxiii.

[53] *On the Venereal Disease,* p. 4.

[54] Cullen's *Elements of Practical Medicine,* pt. 2, i, 3, ch. vii.

whooping-cough were not a disease that has only a partial similarity to the measles, that is to say, if it had also a cutaneous eruption similar to what the latter possesses. As it is, however, the measles can but preserve a large number from whooping-cough, and that only in the epidemic prevailing at the time.

If, however, the *measles* come in contact with a disease resembling it in its chief symptom, the eruption, it can indisputably remove, and effect a homœopathic cure of the latter. Thus a chronic herpetic eruption was entirely and permanently (homœopathically) cured[55] by the breaking out of the measles. as Kortum[56] observed. An excessively burning miliary rash on the face, neck, and arms, that had lasted six years, and was aggravated by every change of weather, on the invasion of measles assumed the form of a swelling of the surface of the skin; after the measles had run its course the exanthem was cured, and returned no more.[57]

§ 47.

Nothing could teach the physician in a plainer and more convincing manner than the above what kind of artificial morbific agent (medicine) he ought to choose in order to cure in a sure, rapid and permanent manner, conformably with the process that takes place in nature.

---

[55] Or at least that symptom was removed

[56] In *Hufeland's Journal*, xx, 3, p. 50.

[57] Rau, *Ueber d. Werth des hom. Heilv.*, Heidelb., 1824, p. 85.

§ 48.

Neither in the course of nature, as we see from all the above examples, nor by the physician's art, can an existing affection or malady in any one instance be removed by a dissimilar morbific agent, be it ever so strong, but *solely by one that is similar in symptoms and is somewhat stronger,* according to eternal, irrevocable laws of nature, which have not hitherto been recognized.

§ 49.

We should have been able to meet with many more real, natural homœopathic cures of this kind if, on the one hand, the attention of observers had been more directed to them, and, on the other hand, if nature had not been so deficient in helpful homœopathic diseases.

§ 50.

Mighty Nature herself has, as we see, at her command, as instruments for effecting homœopathic cures, little besides the miasmatic diseases of constant character (the itch), measles and smallpox,[58] morbific agents which,[59] as remedies, are either more dangerous to life and more to be dreaded than the disease they are to cure, or of such a kind (like the itch) that, after they have effected the

---

[58] And the exanthematous contagious principle present in the cow-pox lymph.

[59] Namely, smallpox and measles.

cure, they themselves require curing, in order to be eradicated in their turn—both circumstances that make their employment, as homœopathic remedies, difficult, uncertain and dangerous. And how few diseases are there to which man is subject that find their similar remedy in smallpox, measles or itch! Hence, in the course of nature, very few maladies can be cured by these uncertain and hazardous homœopathic remedies, and the cure by their instrumentality is also attended with danger and much difficulty, for this reason, that the doses of these morbific powers cannot be diminished according to circumstances, as doses of medicine can; but the patient afflicted with an analogous malady of long standing must be subjected to the entire dangerous and tedious disease, to the entire disease of smallpox, measles (or itch), which in its turn has to be cured. And yet, as is seen, we can point to some striking homœopathic cures effected by this lucky concurrence, also many incontrovertible proofs of the great, the sole therapeutic law of nature that obtains in them: *Cure by symptom similarity!*

§ 51.

This therapeutic law is rendered obvious to all intelligent minds by these facts, and they are amply sufficient for this end. But, on the other hand, see what advantages man has over crude Nature in her happy-go-lucky operations. How many thousands more of homœopathic morbific agents has not man at his disposal for the relief of his suffering fellow-creatures in the medicinal substances universally distributed throughout creation!

In them he has producers of disease of all possible varieties of action, for all the innumerable, for all conceivable
and inconceivable natural diseases, to which they can
render homœopathic aid—morbific agents (medicinal
substances), whose power, when their remedial employment is completed, being overcome by the vital force,
disappears spontaneously without requiring a second
course of treatment for its extirpation, like the itch—
artificial morbific agents, which the physician can atten-
uate, subdivide and potentize almost to an infinite extent,
and the dose of which he can diminish to such a degree
that they shall remain only slightly stronger than the
similar natural disease they are employed to cure; so that
in this incomparable method of cure, there is no necessity
for any violent attack upon the organism for the eradication of even an inveterate disease of old standing; the
cure by this method takes place by only a gentle, imperceptible and yet often rapid transition from the tormenting natural disease to the desired state of permanent
health.

§ 52.

There are but two principal methods of cure: the one
based only on accurate observation of nature, on careful
experimentation and pure experience, the homœopathic
(before we never designedly used) and a second which
does not do this, the heteropathic or allopathic. Each
opposes the other, and only he who does not know either
can hold the delusion that they can ever approach each
other or even become united, or to make himself so
ridiculous as to practice at one time homœopathically at

another allopathically, according to the pleasure of the patient; a practice which may be called criminal treason against divine homœopathy.

§ 53.

The true mild cures take place only according to the homœopathic method, which, as we have found (§ § 7-25) by experience and deduction, is unquestionably the proper one by which through art the quickest, most certain and most permanent cures are obtained since this healing art rests upon an eternal infallible law of nature.

The pure homœopathic healing art is the only correct method, the one possible to human art, the straightest way to cure, as certain as that there is but one straight line between two given points.

§ 54.

The allopathic method of treatment utilized many things against disease, but usually only improper ones (allœa) and ruled for ages in different forms called systems. Every one of these, following each other from time to time and differing greatly each from the other, honored itself with the name of Rational Medicine.[60]

Every builder of such a system cherished the haughty estimation of himself that he was able to penetrate into

---

[60]As if in the establishment of a science, based only on observation of nature and pure experiment and experience idle speculation and scholastic vaporings could have a place.

the inner nature of life of the healthy as well as of the sick and clearly to recognize it and accordingly gave the prescription *which* noxious matter [61] should be banished from the sick man, and *how* to banish it in order to restore him to health, all this according to empty assumptions and arbitrary suppositions without honestly questioning nature and listening without prejudice to the voice of experience. Diseases were held to be conditions that reappeared pretty much in the same manner. Most systems gave, therefore, names to their imagined disease pictures and classified them, every system differently. To medicines were ascribed actions which were supposed to cure these abnormal conditions. (Hence the numerous text books on Materia Medica.[62])

§ 55.

Soon, however, the public became convinced that the sufferings of the sick increased and heightened with the introduction of every one of these systems and methods

---

[61] Up to the most recent times what is curable in sickness was supposed to be a material that had to be removed since no one could conceive of a dynamic effect (§11 note) of morbific agencies, such as medicines exercise upon the life of the animal organism.

[62] To fill the measure of self infatuation to overflowing here were mixed (very learnedly) constantly more, indeed, many different medicines in so-called prescriptions to be administered in frequent and large doses and thereby the precious, easily-destroyed human life was endangered in the hands of these perverted ones. Especially so with seton, venesection, emetics, purgatives, plasters, fontanelles and cauterization.

of cure if followed exactly. Long ago these allopathic physicians would have been left had it not been for the palliative relief obtained at times from empirically discovered remedies whose almost instantaneous flattering action is apparent to the patient and this to some extent served to keep up their credit.

§ 56.

By means of this palliative (antipathic, enantipathic) method, introduced according to Galen's teaching "Contraria contrariis" for seventeen centuries, the physicians hitherto could hope to win confidence while they deluded with almost instantaneous amelioration. But how fundamentally unhelpful and hurtful this method of treatment is (in diseases not running a rapid course) we shall see in what follows. It is certainly the only one of the modes of treatment adopted by the allopaths that had any manifest relation to a portion of the sufferings caused by the natural disease; but what kind of relation? Of a truth the very one (the exact contrary of the right one) that ought carefully to be avoided if we would not delude and make a mockery of the patient affected with a chronic disease.[63]

---

[63] A third mode of employing medicines in diseases has been attempted to be created by means of *Isopathy*, as it is called— that is to say, a method of curing a given disease by the same contagious principle that produces it. But even granting this could be done, yet, after all, seeing that the virus is given to the patient highly potenized, and, consequently, in an altered condi-

§ 57.

In order to carry into practice this antipathic method, the ordinary physician gives, for a single troublesome symptom from among the many other symptoms of the disease which he passes by unheeded, a medicine concerning which it is known that it produces the exact opposite of the morbid symptom sought to be subdued, from which he can expect the speediest (palliative)

---

tion, the cure is effected only by opposing a *simillimum* to a *simillimum*.

To attempt to cure by means of the very same morbific potency (per Idem) contradicts all normal human understanding and hence all experience. Those who first brought Isopathy to notice, probably thought of the benefit which mankind received from cowpox vaccination by which the vaccinated individual is protected against future smallpox infection and as it were cured in advance. But both, cowpox and smallpox are only similar, in no way the same disease. In many respects they differ, namely in the more rapid course and mildness of cowpox and especially in this, that it is never contagious to man by mere nearness. Universal vaccination put an end to all epidemics of that deadly fearful smallpox to such an extent that the present generation does no longer possess a clear conception of the former frightful smallpox plague.

Moreover, in this way, undoubtedly, certain diseases peculiar to animals may give us remedies and medicinal potencies for very similar important human diseases and thus happily enlarge our stock of homœopathic remedies.

But to use a human morbific matter (a Psorin taken from the itch in man) as a remedy for the same human itch or for evils arisen therefrom is —— ?

Nothing can result from this but trouble and aggravation of the disease.

relief. He gives large doses of opium, for pains of all sorts, because this drug soon benumbs the sensibility, and administers the same remedy for diarrhœas, because it speedily puts a stop to the peristaltic motion of the intestinal canal and makes it insensible; and also for sleeplessness, because opium rapidly produces a stupefied, comatose sleep; he gives purgatives when the patient has suffered long from constipation and costiveness; he causes the burnt hand to be plunged into cold water, which, from its low degree of temperature, seems instantaneously to remove the burning pain, as if by magic; he puts the patient who complains of chilliness and deficiency of vital heat into warm baths, which warm him immediately; he makes him who is suffering from prolonged debility drink wine, whereby he is instantly enlivened and refreshed; and in like manner he employs other opposite (antipathic) remedial means, but he has very few besides those just mentioned, as it is only of very few substances that some peculiar (primary) action is known to the ordinary medical school.

§ 58.

If, in estimating the value of this mode of employing medicines, we should even pass over the circumstance that it is *an extremely faulty symptomatic treatment* (v. note to § 7), wherein the practitioner devotes his attention in a merely *one-sided manner to a single symptom*, consequently to only a small part of the whole, whereby relief for the totality of the disease, which is what the patient desires, cannot evidently be expected,—we must, on the other hand, demand of experience if, in one single case where such antipathic employment of medicine was made use of in a chronic or persisting affection, after the transient amelioration there did not ensue an increased aggravation of the symptom which was subdued at first in a palliative manner, an aggravation, indeed, of the whole disease? And every attentive observer will agree that, after such short antipathic amelioration, aggravation follows *in every case without exception,* although the ordinary physician is in the habit of giving his patient another explanation of this subsequent aggravation, and ascribes it to malignancy of the original disease, now for the first time showing itself, or to the occurrence of quite a new disease.[64]

---

[64] Little as physicians have hitherto been in the habit of observing accurately, the aggravation that so certainly follows such palliative treatment could not altogether escape their notice. A striking example of this is to be found in J. H. Schulze's *Diss. qua corporis humani momentanearum alterationum specimina quædam expenduntur,* Halæ, 1741, §28. Willis bears testimony to something similar (*Pharm. rat.,* §7, cap. i, p. 298) : "Opiata dolores atrocissimos plerumque sedant atque indolentiam—procurant, eamque—aliquamdiu et pro stato quodam tempore continuant, quo spatio elapso dolores mox recrudescunt et brevi ad solitam ferociam augentur." And also at page 295 : "Exactis opii viribus illico redeunt tormina, nec atrocitatem suam remittunt, nisi dum ab eodem pharmaco rursus incantuntur." In like manner J. Hunter (*On the Venereal Disease,* p. 13) says that wine and cordials given to the weak increase the action without giving real strength, and the powers of the body are afterwards sunk proportionally as they have been raised, by which nothing can be gained, but a great deal may be lost.

§ 59.

Important symptoms of persistent diseases *have never* yet been treated with such palliative, antagonistic remedies, without the opposite state, a relapse—indeed, a palpable aggravation of the malady—occurring a few hours afterwards. For a persistent tendency to sleepiness during the day the physician prescribed coffee, whose primary action is to enliven; and when it had exhausted its action the day-somnolence increased—for frequent waking at night he gave in the evening, without heeding the other symptoms of the disease, opium, which by virtue of its primary action produced the same night (stupefied, dull) sleep, but the subsequent nights were still more sleepless than before—to chronic diarrhœas he opposed, without regarding the other morbid signs, the same opium, whose primary action is to constipate the bowels, and after a transient stoppage of the diarrhœa it subsequently became all the worse—violent and frequently recurring pains of all kinds he could suppress with opium for but a short time; they then always returned in greater, often intolerable severity, or some much worse affection came in their stead. For nocturnal cough of long standing the ordinary physician knew no better than to administer opium, whose primary action is to suppress every irritation; the cough would then perhaps cease the first night, but during the subsequent nights it would be still more severe, and if it were again and again suppressed by this palliative in increased doses, fever and nocturnal perspiration were added to the disease—weakness of the bladder, with consequent retention of urine, was sought to be conquered by the antipathic work of cantharides to stimulate the urinary passages, whereby evacuation of the urine was certainly at first effected, but thereafter the bladder becomes less capable of stimulation and less able to contract, and paralysis of the bladder is imminent—with large doses of purgative drugs and laxative salts, which excite the bowels to frequent evacuation, it was sought to remove a chronic tendency to constipation, but in the secondary action the bowels became still more confined;—the ordinary physician seeks to remove chronic debility by the administration of wine, which, however, stimulates only in its primary action, and hence the forces sink all the lower in the secondary action;—by bitter substances and heating condiments he tries to strengthen and warm the chronically weak and cold stomach, but in the secondary action of these palliatives, which are stimulating in their primary action only, the stomach becomes yet more inactive;—long-standing deficiency of vital heat and chilly disposition ought surely to yield to prescriptions of warm baths, but still more weak, cold, and chilly do the patients subsequently become;—severely burnt parts feel instantaneous alleviation from the application of cold water, but the burning pain afterwards increases to an incredible degree, and the inflammation spreads and rises to a still greater height;[a]—by means of the sternutatory remedies that provoke a secretion of mucus, coryza with stoppage of the nose of long standing is sought to be removed, but it escapes observation that the disease is aggravated all the more by these antagonistic remedies (in their secondary action), and the nose becomes still

---

[a] Vide Introduction.

more stopped;—by electricity and galvanism, which in their primary action greatly stimulate muscular action, chronically weak and almost paralytic limbs were soon excited to more active movements, but the consequence (the secondary action) was complete deadening of all muscular irritability and complete paralysis;—by venesections it was attempted to remove chronic determination of blood to the head, but they were always followed by greater congestion;—ordinary medical practitioners know nothing better with which to treat the paralytic torpor of the corporeal and mental organs, conjoined with unconsciousness, which prevails in many kinds of typhus, than with large doses of valerian, because this is one of the most powerful medicinal agents for causing animation and increasing the motor faculty; in their ignorance, however, they knew not that this action is only a primary action, and that the organism, after that is passed, most certainly falls back, in the secondary (antagonistic) action, into still greater stupor and immobility, that is to say, into paralysis of the mental and corporeal organs (and death); they did not see, that the very diseases they supplied most plentifully with valerian, which is in such cases an oppositely acting, antipathic remedy, most infallibly terminated fatally. The old school physician rejoices [65] that he is able to reduce for several hours the velocity of the small rapid pulse in cachectic patients with the very first dose of uncombined purple foxglove (which in its *primary* action makes the pulse slower); its rapidity, however, soon returns; repeated, and now increased doses effect an ever smaller

---

[65] Vide Hufeland, in his pamphlet, *die Homöopatie,* p. 20.

diminution of its rapidity, and at length none at all—
indeed in the *secondary* action the pulse becomes uncountable; sleep, appetite and strength depart, and a
speedy death is *invariably* the result, or else insanity
ensues. How often, in one word, the disease is aggravated, or something even worse is effected by the secondary action of such antagonistic (antipathic) remedies,
the old school with its false theories does not perceive,
but experience teaches it in a terrible manner.

§ 60.

If these ill-effects are produced, as may very naturally
be expected from the antipathic employment of medicines, the ordinary physician imagines he can get over
the difficulty by giving, at each renewed aggravation, a
stronger dose of the remedy, whereby an equally transient suppression [66] is effected; and as there then is a still

---

[66] All usual palliatives given for the suffering of the sick have
(as is seen here) as after effects an increase of the same suffering and the older physicians had to repeat them in ever stronger
doses in order to achieve a similar modification, which, however,
was never permanent and never sufficient to prevent an increased
recurrence of the ailment. But Brousseau, who twenty-five years
before contented against the senseless mixing of different drugs
in prescriptions and thereby ended its reign in France, (for which
mankind is grateful to him) introduced his so-called physiological system (without taking note of the homœopathic method
then already established), a method of treatment, while effec-
tively lessening and permanently preventing the return of all the
sufferings, was applicable to all diseases of mankind; a thing
that the palliatives then in use were not capable of affecting.
Being unable to heal disease with mild innocent remedies and

greater necessity for giving ever-increasing quantities of the palliative there ensues either another more serious

---

thus establish health, Brousseau found *the easier way* to quiet the sufferings of patients more and more at the cost of their life and at last to extinguish life wholly—a method of treatment that, alas, seemed sufficient to his contemporaries. In the degree that the patient retains his strength will his ailments be apparent and the more intensely will he feel his pains. He moans and groans and cries out and calls for help more and more vociferously so that the physician cannot come any too soon to give relief. Brousseau needed only to depress the vital force, to lessen it more and more and behold, the more frequently the patient was bled, the more leeches and cupping glasses sucked out the vital fluid (for the innocent irreplaceable blood was according to him responsible for almost all ailments). In the same proportion the patient lost strength to feel pain or to express his aggravated condition by violent complaint and gestures. The patient appears more quiet in proportion as he grows weaker, the bystanders rejoice in his apparent improvement, ready to return to the same measures on the renewal of his sufferings—be they spasms, suffocation, fears or pain, for they had so beautifully quieted him before and gave promise of further ease. In diseases of long duration and when the patient retained some strength, he was deprived of food, put on a "hunger diet," in order to depress life so much more successfully and inhibit the restless states. The debilitated patient feels unable to protest against further similar measures of blood-letting leeches, vesication, warm baths and so forth to refuse their employment. That death must follow such *frequently repeated* reduction and exhaustion of the vital energy is not noticed by the patient, already robbed of all consciousness, and the relatives, blinded by the improvement even of the last sufferings of the patient by means of blood letting and warm baths, cannot understand and are surprised when the patient quietly slips away.

"But God knows the patient on his bed of sickness was not

disease or frequently incurability, even danger of life and death itself, *but never a cure* of a disease of considerable or of long standing.

---

treated with violence, for the prick of a small lancet is not really painful and the gum Arabic solution (Eau de Gourme, almost the only medicine that Brousseau used) was mild in taste and without apparent action—the bite of the leeches insignificant and the blood letting by the physician done quietly while the lukewarm baths could only soothe, hence the disease from the very start must have been fatal, so that the patient, notwithstanding all efforts of the physician, had to leave the earth." In this way the relatives, and especially the heirs of the dear departed, consoled themselves.

The physicians in Europe and elsewhere accepted *this convenient treatment of all diseases* according to a single rule, since it saved them from all further thinking (the most laborious of all work under the sun). They only had to take care "to assuage the pangs of conscience and console themselves that they were not the originators of this system and this method of treatment, that all the other thousands of Brousseauists did the same and that possibly everything would cease with death anyway as was taught by their master." In this way many thousand physicians were miserably misled to shed (with cold heart) the warm blood of their patients that were capable of cure and thereby rob millions of men gradually of their life according to Brousseau's method, more than fell on Napoleon's battlefields. Was it perhaps necessary by the disposition of God for that system of Brousseau which destroyed medically the life of curable patients to precede homœopathy in order to open the eyes of the world to the only true science and art of medicine, homœopathy, in which all curable patients find health and new life when this most difficult of all arts is practised by an indefatigable discriminating physician in a pure and conscientious manner?

§ 61.

Had physicians been capable of reflecting on the sad results of the antagonistic employment of medicines, they had long since discovered the grand truth, THAT THE TRUE RADICAL HEALING ART MUST BE FOUND IN THE EXACT OPPOSITE OF SUCH AN ANTIPATHIC TREATMENT OF THE SYMPTOMS OF DISEASE; they would have become convinced, that as a medicinal action antagonistic to the symptoms of the disease (an antipathically employed medicine) is followed by only transient relief, and after that is passed, by invariable aggravation, the converse of that procedure, *the homœopathic employment of medicines* according to similarity of symptoms, must effect a permanent and perfect cure, if at the same time the opposite of their large doses, the most minute doses, are exhibited. But neither the obvious aggravation that ensued from their antipathic treatment, nor the fact that no physician ever effected a permanent cure of diseases of considerable or of long standing unless some homœopathic medicinal agent was accidentally a chief ingredient in his prescription, nor yet the circumstance that all the rapid and perfect cures that nature ever performed (§ 46), were always effected by the supervention upon the old disease of one of a *similar* character, ever taught them, during such a long series of centuries, this truth, the knowledge of which can alone conduce to the benefit of the sick.

§ 62.

But on what this pernicious result of the palliative, antipathic treatment and the efficacy of the reverse, the homœopathic treatment, depend, is explained by the following facts, deduced from manifold observations, which no one before me perceived, though they are so very palpable and so very evident, and are of such infinite importance to the healing art.

§ 63.

Every agent that acts upon the vitality, every medicine, deranges more or less the vital force, and causes a certain alteration in the health of the individual for a longer or a shorter period. This is termed *primary action*. Although a product of the medicinal and vital powers conjointly, it is principally due to the former power. To its action our vital force endeavors to oppose its own energy. This resistent action is a property, is indeed an automatic action of our life-preserving power, which goes by the name of *secondary action* or *counteraction*.

§ 64.

During the primary action of the artificial morbific agents (medicines) on our healthy body, as seen in the following examples, our vital force seems to conduct itself merely in a passive (receptive) manner, and appears, so to say, compelled to permit the impressions of the artificial power acting from without to take place in it and thereby alter its state of health; it then, however, appears to rouse itself again, as it were, and to develop (A) the exact opposite condition of health (*counteraction, secondary action*) to this effect (*primary action*) produced upon it, if there be such an opposite, and that in as great a degree as was the effect (*primary action*) of the artificial morbific or medicinal agent on it, and proportionate to its own energy;—or (B) if there be not in nature a state exactly the opposite of the primary action, it appears to endeavor to indifferentiate itself, that is, to make its superior power available in the extinction of the change wrought in it from without (by the medicine), in the place of which it substitutes its normal state (*secondary action, curative action*):

§ 65.

Examples of (A) are familiar to all. A hand bathed in hot water is at first much warmer than the other hand that has not been so treated (primary action); but when it is withdrawn from the hot water and again thoroughly dried, it becomes in a short time cold, and at length much colder than the other (secondary action). A person heated by violent exercise (primary action) is afterwards affected with chilliness and shivering (secondary action). To one who was yesterday heated by drinking much wine (primary action), today every breath of air feels too cold (counter-action of the organism, secondary action). An arm that has been kept long in very cold water is at first much paler and colder (primary action) than the other; but removed from the cold water and dried, it subsequently becomes not only warmer than the other, but even hot, red and inflamed (secondary action, reaction of the vital force). Excessive vivacity follows the use of strong coffee (primary action), but sluggishness and drowsiness remain for a long time afterwards (reaction, secondary action), if this be not always again removed for a short time by imbibing fresh supplies of coffee (palliative). After the profound stupefied sleep caused by opium (primary action), the following night will be all the more sleepless (reaction, secondary action). After the constipation produced by opium (primary action), diarrhœa ensues (secondary action); and after purgation with medicines that irritate the bowels, constipation of several days' duration ensues (secondary action). And in like manner it always happens, after the primary action of a medicine that produces in large doses a great change in the health of a healthy person, that its exact opposite, when, as has been observed, there is actually such a thing, is produced in the secondary action by our vital force.

§ 66.

An obvious antagonistic secondary action, however, is, as may readily be conceived, not to be noticed from the action of quite minute homœopathic doses of the deranging agents on the healthy body. A small dose of every one of them certainly produces a primary action that is perceptible to a sufficiently attentive observer; but the living organism employs against it only so much reaction (secondary action) as is necessary for the restoration of the normal condition.

§ 67.

These incontrovertible truths, which spontaneously offer themselves to our notice in nature and experience, explain to us the beneficial action that takes place under homœo-pathic treatment; whilst, on the other hand, they demonstrate the perversity of the antipathic and palliative treatment of diseases with antagonistically acting medicines.[67]

---

[67] Only in the most urgent cases, where danger to life and imminent death allow no time for the action of a homœopathic remedy—not hours, sometimes not even quarter-hours, and scarcely minutes—in sudden accidents occurring to previously healthy individuals—for example, in asphyxia and suspended animation from lightning, from suffocation, freezing, drowning, etc.—is it admissible and judicious, at all events as a preliminary measure, to stimulate the irritability and sensibility (the physical life) with a palliative, as, for instance, with gentle electrical shocks, with clysters of strong coffee, with a stimulating odor, gradual application of heat, etc. When this stimulation is effected, the play of the vital organs again goes on in its former healthy manner, for there is here no disease* to be removed, but merely an obstruction and suppression of the healthy vital force. To this category belong various antidotes to sudden poisonings: alkalies for mineral acids, hepar sulphuris for metallic poisons, coffee and camphor (and ipecacuanha) for poisoning by opium, etc.

It does not follow that a homœopathic medicine has been ill selected for a case of disease because some of the medicinal symptoms are only antipathic to some of the less important and minor symptoms of the disease; if only the others, the stronger, well-marked (characteristic), and peculiar symptoms of the disease are covered and matched by the same medicine with similarity of symptoms—that is to say, overpowered, destroyed and extinguished; the few opposite symptoms also disappear of themselves after the expiry of the term of action of the medicament, without retarding the cure in the least.

---

* And yet the new sect that mixes the two systems appeals (though in vain) to this observation, in order that they may

§ 68.

In *homœopathic* cures experience teaches us that from the uncommonly small doses of medicine (§§ 275-287) required in this method of treatment, which are just sufficient, by the similarity of their symptoms, to overpower and remove from the sensation of the life principle the similar natural disease, there certainly remains, after the destruction of the latter, at first a certain amount of medicinal disease alone in the organism, but, on account of the extraordinary minuteness of the dose, it is so transient, so slight, and disappears so rapidly of its own accord, that the vital force has no need to employ, against this small artificial derangement of its health, any more considerable reaction than will suffice to elevate its present state of health up to the healthy point—that is, than will suffice to effect complete recovery, for which, after the extinction of the previous morbid derangement but little effort is required (§ 64, B).

§ 69.

In the antipathic (palliative) mode of treatment, however, precisely the reverse of this takes place. The medicinal symptom which the physician opposes to the disease

---

have an excuse for encountering everywhere such exceptions to the general rule in diseases, and to justify their convenient employment of allopathic palliatives, and of other injurious allopathic trash besides, solely for the sake of sparing themselves the trouble of seeking for the suitable homœopathic remedy for each case of disease—and thus conveniently appear as homœopathic physicians, without being such. But their performances are on a par with the system they pursue; they are corrupting.

symptom (for example, the insensibility and stupefaction caused by opium in its primary action to acute pain) is certainly not alien, not wholly allopathic to the latter; there is a manifest relation of the medicinal symptom to the disease symptom, but it is the *reverse* of what should be; it is here intended that the annihilation of the disease symptom shall be effected by an *opposite* medicinal symptom, which is nevertheless impossible. No doubt the antipathically chosen medicine touches precisely the same diseased point in the organism as the homœopathic medicine chosen on account of the similar affection it produces; but the former covers but lightly the opposite symptom of the disease only as an opposite, and makes it unobservable to our life principle for a short time only, so that in the first period of the action of the antagonistic palliative the vital force perceives nothing disagreeable from either of the two (neither from the disease symptom nor from the medicinal symptom), as they seem both to have mutually removed and dynamically neutralized one another as it were (for example, the stupefying power of opium does this to the pain). In the first minutes the vital force feels quite well, and perceives neither the stupefaction of the opium nor the pain of the disease. But as the antagonistic medicinal symptom cannot (as in the homœopathic treatment) occupy the place of the morbid derangement present in the organism in the sensation of the life principle as a *similar, stronger* (artificial) disease, and cannot, therefore like a homœopathic medicine, affect the vital force with a similar artificial disease, so as to be able to step into the place of the original natural morbid derangement, the palliative medicine must, as a thing totally differing from, and the opposite of the disease derangement, leave the latter uneradicated; it renders it, as before said, by a semblance of dynamic neutralization,[68] at first unfelt by the vital force, but, like every medicinal disease, it is soon spontaneously extinguished, and not only leaves the disease behind, just as it was, but compels the vital force (as it must, like all palliatives, be given in large doses in order to effect the apparent removal) to produce an opposite condition (§§ 63, 64) to this palliative medicine, the reverse of the medicinal action, consequently the analogue of the still present, undestroyed, natural morbid derangement, which is necessarily strengthened and increased [69] by this addition

---

[68] In the living human being no permanent neutralization of contrary or antagonistic sensations can take place, as happens with substances of opposite qualities in the chemical laboratory, where, for instance, sulphuric acid and potash unite to form a perfectly different substance, a neutral salt, which is now no longer either acid or alkali, and is not decomposed even by heat. Such amalgamations and thorough combinations to form something permanently neutral and indifferent do not, as has been said, ever take place with respect to dynamic impressions of an antagonistic nature in our sensific apparatus. Only a semblance of neutralization and mutual removal occurs in such cases at first, but the antagonistic sensations do not permanently remove one another. The tears of the mourner will be dried for but a short time by a laughable play; the jokes are, however, soon forgotten, and his tears then flow still more abundantly than before.

[69] Plain as this proposition is, it has been misunderstood, and in opposition to it some have asserted "that the palliative in its secondary action, which would then be similar to the disease present, must be capable of curing just as well as a homœopathic medicine does by its primary action." But they did not reflect

(reaction against the palliative) produced by the vital force. *The disease symptom* (this single part of the disease) *consequently becomes worse after the term of the action of the palliative has expired; worse in proportion to the magnitude of the dose of the palliative.* Accordingly (to keep to the same example) the larger the dose of opium given to allay the pain, so much the more does the pain increase beyond its original intensity as soon as the opium has exhausted its action.[70]

§ 70.

From what has been already adduced we cannot fail to draw the following inferences:

That everything of a really morbid character and which ought to be cured that the physician can discover in diseases consists solely of the sufferings of the patient, and the sensible alterations in

---

that the secondary action is not a product of the medicine, but invariably of the antagonistically acting vital force of the organism; that therefore this secondary action resulting from the vital force on the employment of a palliative is a state similar to the symptoms of the disease which the palliative left uneradicated, and which the reaction of the vital force against the palliative consequently increased still more.

[70] As when in a dark dungeon, where the prisoner could with difficulty recognize objects close to him, alcohol is suddenly lighted, everything is instantly illuminated in a most consolatory manner to the unhappy wretch; but when it is extinguished, the brighter the flame was previously the blacker is the night which now envelopes him, and renders everything about him much more difficult to be seen than before.

his health, in a word, solely of the totality of the symptoms, by means of which the disease demands the medicine requisite for its relief; whilst, on the other hand, every internal cause attributed to it, every occult quality or imaginary material morbific principle, is nothing but an idle dream;

That this derangement of the state of health, which we term disease, can only be converted into health by another revolution effected in the state of health by means of medicines, whose sole curative power, consequently, can only consist in altering man's state of health—that is to say, in a peculiar excitation of morbid symptoms, and is learned with most distinctness and purity by testing them on the healthy body;

That, according to all experience, a natural disease can never be cured by medicines that possess the power of producing in the healthy individual an alien morbid state (dissimilar morbid symptoms) *differing* from that of the disease to be cured (never, therefore, by an allopathic mode of treatment), and that even in nature no cure ever takes place in which an inherent disease is removed, annihilated and cured by the addition of another disease dissimilar to it, be the new one ever so strong;

That, moreover, all experience proves that, by means of medicines which have a tendency to produce in the healthy individual an artificial morbid symptom, *antagonistic* to the single symptom of disease sought to be cured, the cure of a long-standing affection will never be effected, but merely a very transient alleviation, always followed by its aggravation; and that, in a word, this antipathic and merely palliative treatment in long-standing diseases of a serious character is absolutely inefficacious;

That, however, the third and only other possible mode of treatment (the *homœopathic*), in which there is employed *for the totality of the symptoms* of a natural disease a medicine capable of producing the most similar symptoms possible in the healthy individual, given in suitable dose, is the only efficacious remedial method whereby diseases, which are purely dynamic deranging irritations of the vital force, are overpowered, and being thus easily, perfectly and permanently extinguished, must necessarily cease to exist. This is brought about by means of the stronger similar deranging irritations of the homœopathic medicine in the sensation of the life principle. For this mode of procedure we have the example of unfettered Nature herself, when to an old disease there is added a new one similar to the first, whereby the new one is rapidly and forever annihilated and cured.

§ 71.

As it is now no longer a matter of doubt that the diseases of mankind consist merely of groups of certain symptoms, and may be annihilated and transformed into health by medicinal substances, but only by such as are capable of artificially producing similar morbid symptoms (and such is the process in all genuine cures), hence the operation of curing is comprised in the three following points:

I. How is the physician to ascertain what is necessary to be known in order to cure the disease?

II. How is he to gain a knowledge of the instruments adapted for the cure of the natural disease, the pathogenetic powers of the medicines?

III. What is the most suitable method of employing these artificial morbific agents (medicines) for the cure of natural disease?

§ 72.

With respect to the first point, the following will serve as a general preliminary view. The diseases to which man is liable are either rapid morbid processes of the abnormally deranged vital force, which have a tendency to finish their course more or less quickly, but always in a moderate time—these are termed *acute* diseases;—or they are diseases of such a character that, with small, often imperceptible beginnings, dynamically derange the living organism, each in its own peculiar manner, and cause it gradually to deviate from the healthy condition, in such a way that the automatic life energy, called vital force, whose office is to preserve the health, only opposes to them at the commencement and during their progress imperfect, unsuitable, useless resistance, but is unable of

11

itself to extinguish them, but must helplessly suffer (them to spread and) itself to be ever more and more abnormally deranged, until at length the organism is destroyed; these are termed *chronic* diseases. They are caused by dynamic infection with a chronic miasm.

§ 73.

As regards acute diseases, they are either of such a kind as attack human beings individually, *the exciting cause* being injurious influences to which they were particularly exposed. Excesses in food, or an insufficient supply of it, severe physical impressions, chills, overheatings, dissipation, strains, etc., or physical irritations, mental emotions, and the like, are exciting causes of such acute febrile affections; in reality, however, they are generally only a transient explosion of latent psora, which spontaneously returns to its dormant state if the acute diseases were not of too violent a character and were soon quelled. Or they are of such a kind as attack several persons at the same time, here and there (*sporadically*), by means of meteoric or telluric influences and injurious agents, the susceptibility for being morbidly affected by which is possessed by only a few persons at one time. Allied to these are those diseases in which many persons are attacked with very similar sufferings from the same cause (*epidemically*); these diseases generally become infectious (*contagious*) when they prevail among thickly congregated masses of human beings. Thence arise fevers,[71] in each instance of a peculiar

---

[71] The homœopathic physician, who does not entertain the foregone conclusions devised by the ordinary school (who have fixed

nature, and, because the cases of disease have an identical origin, they set up in all those they affect an identical morbid process, which when left to itself terminates in a moderate period of time in death or recovery. The calamities of war, inundations and famine are not infrequently their exciting causes and producers—sometimes they are peculiar *acute miasms* which recur in the same manner (hence known by some traditional name), which either attack persons but once in a lifetime, as the small-pox, measles, whooping-cough, the ancient, smooth, bright red scarlet fever[72] of Sydenham, the mumps, etc., or such as recur frequently in pretty much the same manner, the plague of the Levant, the yellow fever of the sea-coast, the Asiatic cholera, etc.

---

upon a few names of such fevers, besides which mighty nature dare not produce any others, so as to admit of their treating these diseases according to some fixed method), does not acknowledge the names gaol fever, bilious fever, typhus fever, putrid fever, nervous fever or mucous fever, but treats them each according to their several peculiarities.

[72] Subsequently to the year 1801 a kind of purpura miliaris (*roodvonk*), which came from the West, was by physicians confounded with the scarlet fever, notwithstanding that they exhibited totally different symptoms, that the latter found its prophylactic and curative remedy in belladonna, the former in aconite, and that the former was generally merely sporadic, while the latter was invariably epidemic. Of late years it seems as if the two occasionally joined to form an eruptive fever of a peculiar kind, for which neither the one nor yet the other remedy, alone, will be found to be exactly homœopathic.

§ 74.

Among chronic diseases we must still, alas! reckon those so commonly met with, artifically produced in allopathic treatment by the prolonged use of violent heroic medicines in large and increasing doses, by the abuse of calomel, corrosive sublimate, mercurial ointment, nitrate of silver, iodine and its ointments, opium, valerian, cinchona bark and quinine, foxglove, prussic acid, sulphur and sulphuric acid, perennial purgatives,[73] venesections, shedding streams of blood, leeches, issues, setons, etc., whereby the vital energy is sometimes weakened to an unmerciful extent, sometimes, if it do not succumb, gradually abnormally deranged (by each substance in a peculiar manner) in such a way that, in order to maintain life against these inimical and destructive attacks, it must produce a revolution in the organism, and either deprive some part of its irritability and sensibility, or exalt these to an excessive degree, cause dilatation or contraction, relaxation or induration or even total destruction of certain parts, and develop faulty organic alterations here and there in the interior or the exterior (cripple the body internally or externally), in order to preserve the organism from complete destruction of life by the ever-renewed, hostile assaults of such destructive forces.[74]

---

[73] The only possible case of plethora shows itself with the healthy woman, several days before her monthly period, with a feeling of a certain fulness of womb and breasts, but without inflammation.

[74] Among all imaginable methods for the relief of sickness, no greater allopathic, irrational or inappropriate one can be thought

§ 75.

These inroads on human health effected by the allo-pathic non-healing art (more particularly in recent times) are of all chronic diseases the most deplorable, the most

---

of than this Brousseauic, debilitating treatment by means of vene-section and hunger diet, which, for many years, has spread over a large part of the earth. No intelligent man can see in it any-thing medical or medicinally helpful, whereas real medicines, even if chosen blindly and administered to a patient, may at times prove of benefit in a given case of sickness because they may accidentally have been homœopathic to the case. But from venesection, healthy common sense can expect nothing more than certain lessening and shortening of life. It is a sorrowful and wholly groundless fallacy that most and indeed all diseases de-pend on local inflammation. Even for true local inflammation, the most certain and quickest cure is found in medicines capa-ble of taking away dynamically the arterial irritation upon which the inflammation is based and this without the least loss of fluids and strength. Local venesections, even from the affected part, only tend to increase renewed inflammation of these parts. And precisely so it is generally inappropriate, aye, murderous, to take away many pounds of blood from the veins in inflamma-tory fevers, when a few appropriate medicines would dispel this irritated arterial state, driving the hitherto quiet blood to-gether with the disease in a few hours without the least loss of fluids and strength. Such great loss of blood is evidently irre-placeable for the remaining continuance of life, since the organs intended by the Creator for bloodmaking have thereby become so weakened that while they may manufacture blood in the same quantity but not again of the same good quality. And how im-possible is it for this imagined plethora to have been produced in such remarkable rapidity and so to drain it off by frequent venesections when yet an hour before the pulse of this heated patient (before the fever and chill stage) was so quiet. No

incurable; and I regret to add that it is apparently impossible to discover or to hit upon any remedies for their cure when they have reached any considerable height.

§ 76.

Only for natural diseases has the beneficent Deity granted us, in Homœopathy, the means of affording relief; but those devastations and maimings of the human organism exteriorly and interiorly, effected by years frequently, of the unsparing exercise of a false art,[75] with

---

man, no sick person has ever too much blood or too much strength. On the contrary, every sick man lacks strength, otherwise his vital energy would have prevented the development of the disease. Thus it is irrational and cruel to add to this weakened patient a greater, indeed the most serious source of debility that can be imagined. It is a murderous malpractice irrational and cruel based on a wholly groundless and absurd theory instead of taking away his disease which is ever dynamic and only to be removed by dynamic potencies.

[75] If the patient at length succumbs, the practiser of such a treatment is in the habit of pointing out to the sorrowing relatives, at the *post-mortem* examination, these internal organic disfigurements, which are due to his pseudo-art, but which he artfully maintains to be the original incurable disease (see my book, *Die Allöopathic ein Wort der Warnung an Kranke jeder Art,* Leipzig, bei Baumgartner [translated in *Lesser Writings*]). Those deceitful records, the illustrated works on pathological anatomy, exhibit the products of such lamentable bungling. *Deceased people from the country and those from the poor of cities who have died without such bungling with hurtful measures are not opened up through pathological anatomy as a rule.* Such corruption and deformities would not be found in their corpses. From this

its hurtful drugs and treatment, *must be remedied by the vital force itself* (appropriate aid being given for the eradication of any chronic miasm that may happen to be lurking in the background), if it has not already been too much weakened by such mischievous acts, and can devote several years to this huge operation undisturbed. A human healing art, for the restoration to the normal state of those innumerable abnormal conditions so often produced by the allopathic non-healing art, there is not and cannot be.

§ 77.

Those diseases are inappropriately named chronic which persons incur who expose themselves continually to *avoidable* noxious influences, who are in the habit of indulging in injurious liquors or aliments, are addicted to dissipation of many kinds which undermine the health, who undergo prolonged abstinence from things that are necessary for the support of life, who reside in unhealthy localities, especially marshy districts, who are housed in cellars or other confined dwellings, who are deprived of exercise or of open air, who ruin their health by over-exertion of body or mind, who live in a constant state of worry, etc. These states of ill-health, which persons bring upon themselves disappear spontaneously, provided no chronic miasm lurks in the body, under an improved mode of living, and they cannot be called chronic diseases.

---

fact can be judged the value of the evidence drawn from these beautiful illustrations as well as of the honesty of these authors and book makers.

§ 78.

The true natural *chronic* diseases are those that arise from a chronic miasm, which when left to themselves, and unchecked by the employment of those remedies that are specific for them, always go on increasing and growing worse, notwithstanding the best mental and corporeal regimen, and torment the patient to the end of his life with ever aggravated sufferings. These, excepting those produced by medical malpractice (§ 74), are the most numerous and greatest scourges of the human race; for the most robust constitution, the best regulated mode of living and the most vigorous energy of the vital force are insufficient for their eradication.[76]

§ 79.

Hitherto syphilis alone has been to some extent known as such a chronic miasmatic disease, which when uncured ceases only with the termination of life. Sycosis (the condylomatous disease), equally ineradicable by the vital

---

[76] During the flourishing years of youth and with the commencement of regular menstruation joined to a mode of life beneficial to soul, heart and body, they remain unrecognized for years. Those afflicted appear in perfect health to their relatives and acquaintances and the disease that was received by infection or inheritance seems to have wholly disappeared. But in later years, after adverse events and conditions of life, they are sure to appear anew and develop the more rapidly and assume a more serious character in proportion as the vital principle has become disturbed by debilitating passions, worry and care, but especially when disordered by inappropriate medicinal treatment.

force without proper medicinal treatment, was not recognized as a chronic miasmatic disease of a peculiar character, which it nevertheless undoubtedly is, and physicians imagined they had cured it when they had destroyed the growths upon the skin, but the persisting dyscrasia occasioned by it escaped their observation.

§ 80.

Incalculably greater and more important than the two chronic miasms just named, however, is the chronic miasm of psora, which, whilst those two reveal their specific internal dyscrasia, the one by the venereal chancre, the other by the cauliflower-like growths, does also, after the completion of the internal infection òf the whole organism, announce by a peculiar cutaneous eruption, sometimes consisting only of a few vesicles accompanied by intolerable voluptuous tickling itching (and a peculiar odor), the monstrous internal chronic miasm—the psora, the only real *fundamental cause* and producer of all the other numerous, I may say innumerable, forms of disease,"

" I spent twelve years in investigating the source of this incredibly large number of chronic affections, in ascertaining and collecting certain proofs of this great truth, which had remained unknown to all former or contemporary observers, and in discovering at the same time the principal (antipsoric) remedies, which collectively are nearly a match for this thousand-headed monster of disease in all its different developments and forms. I have published my observations on this subject in the book entitled *The Chronic Diseases* (4 vols., Dresden, Arnold. [2nd edit., Düsseldorf, Schaub.]) before I had obtained this knowl-

which, under the names of nervous debility, hysteria, hypochondriasis, mania, melancholia, imbecility, madness, epilepsy and convulsions of all sorts, softening of the bones (*rachitis*), scoliosis and cyphosis, caries, cancer, fungus hæmatodes, neoplasms, gout, hæmorrhoids, jaundice, cyanosis, dropsy, amenorrhœa, hæmorrhage from the stomach, nose, lungs, bladder and womb, of asthma and ulceration of the lungs, of impotence and barrenness, of megrim, deafness, cataract, amaurosis, urinary calculus, paralysis, defects of the senses and pains of thousands of kinds, etc., figure in systematic works on pathology as peculiar, independent diseases.

---

edge I could only teach how to treat the whole number of chronic diseases as isolated, individual maladies, with those medicinal substances whose pure effects had been tested on healthy persons up to that period, so that every case of chronic disease was treated by my disciples according to the group of symptoms it presented, just like an idiopathic disease, and it was often so far cured that sick mankind rejoiced at the extensive remedial treasures already amassed by the new healing art. How much greater cause is there now for rejoicing that the desired goal has been so much more nearly attained, inasmuch as the recently discovered and far more specific homœopathic remedies for chronic affections arising from psora (properly termed antipsoric remedies) and the special instructions for their preparation and employment have been published; and from among them the true physician can now select for his curative agents those whose medicinal symptoms correspond in the most similar (homœopathic) manner to the chronic disease he has to cure; and thus, by the employment of (antipsoric) medicines more suitable for this miasm, he is enabled to render more essential service and almost invariably to effect a perfect cure.

§ 81.

The fact that this extremely ancient infecting agent has gradually passed, in some hundreds of generations, through many millions of human organisms and has thus attained an incredible development, renders it in some measure conceivable how it can now display such innumerable morbid forms in the great family of mankind, particularly when we consider what a number of circumstances[78] contribute to the production of these great varieties of chronic diseases (secondary symptoms of psora), besides the indescribable diversity of men in respect of their congenital corporeal consitutions, so that it is no wonder if such a variety of injurious agencies acting from within and from without and sometimes continually, on such a variety of organisms permeated with the psoric miasm, should produce an innumerable variety of defects, injuries, derangements and sufferings, which have hitherto been treated of in the old pathological works,[79]

---

[78] Some of these causes that exercise a modifying influence on the transformation of psora into chronic diseases manifestly depend sometimes on the climate and the peculiar physical character of the place of abode, sometimes on the very great varieties in the physical and mental training of youth, both of which may have been neglected, delayed or carried to excess, or on their abuse in the business or conditions of life, in the matter of diet and regimen, passions, manners, habits and customs of various kinds.

[79] How many improper ambiguous names do not these works contain, under each of which are included excessively different morbid conditions, which often resemble each other in one single symptom only, as *ague, jaundice, dropsy, consumption, leucor-*

under a number of special *names*, as diseases of an independent character.

---

rhœa, hæmorrhoids, rheumatism, apoplexy, convulsions, hysteria, hypochrondriasis, melancholia, mania, quinsy, palsy, etc., which are represented as diseases of a fixed and unvarying character, and are treated, on account of their name, according to a determinate plan! How can the bestowal of such a name justify an identical medical treatment? And if the treatment is not always to be the same, why make use of an identical name which postulates an identity of treatment? "Nihil sane in artem medicam pestiferum magis unquam irrepsit malum, quam generalia quædam nomina morbis imponere iisque aptare velle generalem quandam medicinam," says Huxham, a man as clear-sighted as he was estimable on account of his conscientiousness (*Op. phys. med.*, tom. i.). And in like manner Fritze laments (*Annalen*, i, p. 80) "that essentially different diseases are designated by the same name." Even those epidemic diseases, which undoubtedly may be propagated *in every separate epidemic* by a peculiar contagious principle which remains unknown to us, are designated, in the old school of medicine, by particular names, just as if they were well-known fixed diseases that invariably recurred under the same form, as *hospital fever, gaol fever, camp fever, putrid fever, bilious fever, nervous fever, mucous fever*, although each epidemic of such roving fevers exhibits itself at every occurrence as another, a *new* disease, such as it has never before appeared in exactly the same form, differing very much, in every instance, in its course, as well as in many of its most striking symptoms and its whole appearance. Each is so far dissimilar to all previous epidemics, whatever names they may bear, that it would be a dereliction of all logical accuracy in our ideas of things were we to give to these maladies, that differ so much among themselves, one of those names we meet with in pathological writings, and treat them all medicinally in conformity with this misused name. The candid Sydenham alone perceived this, when he (*Obs. med.*, cap. ii, De morb. epid.) insists upon the necessity of not considering any epidemic disease as having oc-

§ 82.

Although, by the discovery of that great source of chronic diseases, as also by the discovery of the specific

---

curred before and treating it in the same way as another, since all that occur successively, be they ever so numerous, differ from one another: "Nihil quicquam (opinor,) animum universæ qua patet medicinæ pomœria perlustrantem, tanta admiratione percellet, quam discolor illa et sui plane dissimilis morborum Epidemicorum facies; non tam qua varias ejusdem anni tempestates, quam qua discrepantes diversorum ab invicem annorum constitutiones referunt, ab iisque dependent. Quæ tam aperta prædictorum morborum diversitas tum propriis ac sibi peculiaribus symptomatis, tum etiam medendi ratione, quam hi ab illis disparem prorsus sibi vendicant, satis illucescit. Ex quibus constat morbus hosce, ut ut externa quadantenus specie, et symptomatis aliquot utrisque pariter supervenientibus, convenire paulo incautioribus videantur, re tamen ipsa (si bene adverteris animum), alienæ admodum esse indolis, et distare ut æra lupinis."

From all this it is clear that these useless and misused names of diseases ought to have no influence on the practice of the true physician, who knows that he has to judge of and to cure diseases, not according to the similarity of the name of a single one of their symptoms, but according to the totality of the signs of the individual state of each particular patient, whose affection it is his duty carefully to investigate, but never to give a hypothetical guess at it.

If, however, it is deemed necessary sometimes to make use of names of diseases, in order, when talking about a patient to ordinary persons, to render ourselves intelligible in few words, we ought only to employ them as collective names and tell them, *e. g.*, the patient has *a kind* of St. Vitus's dance, *a kind* of dropsy, *a kind* of typhus, *a kind* of ague; but (in order to do away once for all with the mistaken notions these names give rise to) we should never say he has *the* St. Vitus's dance, *the* typhus, *the* dropsy, *the* ague, as there are certainly no diseases of these and similar names of fixed unvarying character.

homœopathic remedies for the psora, medicine has advanced some steps nearer to a knowledge of the nature of the majority of diseases it has to cure, yet, for settling the indication in each case of chronic (psoric) disease he is called on to cure, the duty of a careful apprehension of its ascertainable symptoms and characteristics is as indispensable for the homœopathic physician as it was before that discovery, as no real cure of this or of other diseases can take place without a strict particular treatment (individualization) of each case of disease—only that in this investigation some difference is to be made when the affection is an acute and rapidly developed disease, and when it is a chronic one; seeing that, in acute disease, the chief symptoms strike us and become evident to the senses more quickly, and hence much less time is requisite for tracing the picture of the disease and much fewer questions are required to be asked,[80] as almost everything is self-evident, than in a chronic disease which has been gradually progressing for several years, in which the symptoms are much more difficult to be ascertained.

§ 83.

This individualizing *examination of a case of disease,* for which I shall only give in this place general directions, of which the practitioner will bear in mind only what is applicable for each individual case, demands of the physician *nothing but freedom from prejudice and*

---

[80] Hence the following directions for investigating the symptoms are only partially applicable for acute diseases.

sound senses, attention in observing and fidelity in tracing the picture of the disease.

§ 84.

The patient details the history of his sufferings; those about him tell what they heard him complain of, how he has behaved and what they have noticed in him; the physician sees, hears, and remarks by his other senses what there is of an altered or unusual character about him. He writes down accurately all that the patient and his friends have told him in the very expressions used by them. Keeping silence himself, he allows them to say all they have to say, and refrains from interrupting them[81] unless they wander off to other matters. The physician advises them at the beginning of the examination to speak slowly, in order that he may take down in writing the important parts of what the speakers say.

§ 85.

He begins a fresh line with every new circumstance mentioned by the patient or his friends, so that the symptoms shall be all ranged separately one below the other. He can thus add to any one, that may at first have been related in too vague a manner, but subsequently more explicitly explained.

---

[81] Every interruption breaks the train of thought of the narrators, and all they would have said at first does not again occur to them in precisely the same manner after that.

§ 86.

When the narrators have finished what they would say of their own accord, the physician then reverts to each particular symptom and elicits more precise information respecting it in the following manner; he reads over the symptoms as they were related to him one by one, and about each of them he inquires for further particulars: *e. g.*, at what period did this symptom occur? Was it previous to taking the medicine he had hitherto been using? Whilst taking the medicine? Or only some days after leaving off the medicine? What kind of pain, what sensation exactly, was it that occurred on this spot? Where was the precise spot? Did the pain occur in fits and by itself, at various times? Or was it continued, without intermission? How long did it last? At what time of the day or night, and in what position of the body was it worst, or ceased entirely? What was the exact nature of this or that event or circumstance mentioned—described in plain words?

§ 87.

And thus the physician obtains more precise information respecting each particular detail, but without ever framing his questions so as to suggest the answer to the patient,[82] so that he shall only have to answer yes or

---

[82] For instance, the physician should not ask, Was not this or that circumstance present? He should never be guilty of making such suggestions, which tend to seduce the patient into giving a false answer and a false account of his symptoms.

no; else he will be misled to answer in the affirmative or negative something untrue, half true, or not strictly correct, either from indolence or in order to please his interrogator, from which a false picture of the disease and an unsuitable mode of treatment must result.

§ 88.

If in these voluntary details nothing has been mentioned respecting several facts or functions of the body or his mental state, the physician asks what more can he told in regard to these parts and these functions, or the state of his disposition or mind;[83] but in doing this he only makes use of general expressions, in order that his informants may be obliged to enter into special details concerning them.

§ 89.

When the patient (for it is on him we have chiefly to rely for a description of his sensations, except in the case of feigned diseases) has by these details, given of his own

---

[83] For example, what is the character of his stools? How does he pass his water? How is it with his day and night sleep? What is the state of his disposition, his humor, his memory? How about the thirst? What sort of taste has he in his mouth? What kinds of food and drink are most relished? What are most repugnant to him? Has each its full natural taste, or some other unusual taste? How does he feel after eating or drinking? Has he anything to tell about the head, the limbs, or the abdomen?

accord and in answer to inquiries, furnished the requisite information and traced a tolerably perfect picture of the disease, the physician is at liberty and obliged (if he feels he has not yet gained all the information he needs) to ask more precise, more special questions.[84]

---

[84] For example, how often are his bowels moved? What is the exact character of the stools? Did the whitish evacuation consist of mucus or fæces? Had he or had he not pains during the evacuation? What was their exact character, and where were they seated? What did the patient vomit? Is the bad taste in the mouth putrid, or bitter, or sour, or what? before or after eating, or during the repast? At what period of the day was it worst? What is the taste of what is eructated? Does the urine only become turbid on standing, or is it turbid when first discharged? What is its color when first emitted? Of what color is the sediment? How does he behave during sleep? Does he whine, moan, talk or cry out in his sleep? Does he start during sleep? Does he snore during inspiration, or during expiration? Does he lie only on his back, or on which side? Does he cover himself well up, or can he not bear the clothes on him? Does he easily awake, or does he sleep too soundly? How does he feel immediately after waking from sleep? How often does this or that symptom occur? what is the cause that produces it each time it occurs? does it come on whilst sitting, lying, standing, or when in motion? only when fasting, or in the morning, or only in the evening, or only after a meal, or when does it usually appear? When did the rigor come on? was it merely a chilly sensation, or was he actually cold at the same time? if so, in what parts? or while feeling chilly, was he actually warm to the touch? was it merely a sensation of cold, without shivering? was he hot without redness of the face? what parts of him were hot to the touch? or did he complain of heat without being hot to the touch? How long did the chilliness last? how long the hot stage? When did the thirst

§ 90.

When the physician has finished writing down these particulars, he then makes a note of what he himself observes in the patient,[85] and ascertains how much of that was peculiar to the patient in his healthy state.

---

come on—during the cold stage? during the heat? or previous to it? or subsequently to it? How great was the thirst, and what was the beverage desired? When did the sweat come on—at the beginning or the end of the heat? or how many hours after the heat? when asleep or when awake? How great was the sweat? was it warm or cold? on what parts? how did it smell? What does he complain of before or during the cold stage? what during the hot stage? what after it? what during or after the sweating stage?

In women, note the character of menstruation and other discharges, etc.

[85] For example, how the patient behaved during the visit—whether he was morose, quarrelsome, hasty, lachrymose, anxious, despairing or sad, or hopeful, calm, etc. Whether he was in a drowsy state or in any way dull of comprehension; whether he spoke hoarsely, or in a low tone, or incoherently, or how otherwise did he talk? what was the color of his face and eyes, and of his skin generally? what degree of liveliness and power was there in his expression and eyes? what was the state of his tongue, his breathing, the smell from his mouth, and his hearing? were his pupils dilated or contracted? how rapidly and to what extent did they alter in the dark and in the light? what was the character of the pulse? what the condition of the abdomen? how moist or hot, how cold or dry to the touch, was the skin of this or that part, or generally? whether he lay with head thrown back, with mouth half or wholly open, with the arms placed above the head, on his back, or in what other position? what effort did he make to raise himself? and anything else in him that may strike the physician as being remarkable.

§ 91.

The symptoms and feelings of the patient during a previous course of medicine do not furnish the pure picture of the disease; but, on the other hand, those symptoms and ailments which he suffered from *before the use of the medicines, or after they had been discontinued for several days,* give the true fundamental idea of the *original* form of the disease, and these especially the physician must take note of. When the disease is of a chronic character, and the patient has been taking medicine up to the time he is seen, the physician may with advantage leave him some days quite without medicine, or in the meantime administer something of an unmedicinal nature and defer to a subsequent period the more precise scrutiny of the morbid symptoms, in order to be able to grasp in their purity the permanent uncontaminated symptoms of the old affection and to form a faithful picture of the disease.

§ 92.

But if it be a disease of a rapid course, and if its serious character admit of no delay, the physician must content himself with observing the morbid condition, altered though it may be by medicines, if he cannot ascertain what symptoms were present before the employment of the medicines,—in order that he may at least form a just apprehension of the complete picture of the disease in its actual condition, that is to say, of the conjoint malady formed by the medicinal and original diseases, which from the use of inappropriate drugs is generally more serious and dangerous than was the original disease, and hence demands prompt and efficient aid; and by thus tracing out the complete picture of the disease he will be enabled to combat it with a suitable homœopathic remedy, so that the patient shall not fall a sacrifice to the injurious drugs he has swallowed.

§ 93.

If the disease has been brought on a short time, or, in the case of a chronic affection, a considerable time previously, by some obvious cause, then the patient—or his friends when questioned privately—will mention it either spontaneously or when carefully interrogated.[86]

§ 94.

While inquiring into the state of chronic diseases, the particular circumstances of the patient with regard to his

---

[86] Any causes of a disgraceful character, which the patient or his friends do not like to confess, at least not voluntarily, the physician must endeavor to elicit by skilfully framing his questions, or by private information. To these belong poisoning or attempted suicide, onanism, indulgence in ordinary or unnatural debauchery, excesses in wine, cordials, punch and other ardent beverages, or coffee,—over-indulgence in eating generally, or in some particular food of a hurtful character,—infection with venereal disease or itch, unfortunate love, jealousy, domestic infelicity, worry, grief on account of some family misfortune, ill-usage, balked revenge, injured pride, embarrassment of a pecuniary nature, superstitious fear,—hunger,—or an imperfection in the private parts, a rupture, a prolapsus, and so forth.

ordinary occupations, his usual mode of living and diet, his domestic situation, and so forth, must be well considered and scrutinized, to ascertain what there is in them that may tend to produce or to maintain disease, in order that by their removal the recovery may be promoted.[87]

§ 95.

In chronic diseases the investigation of the signs of disease above mentioned, and of all others, must be pursued as carefully and circumstantially as possible, and the most minute peculiarities must be attended to, partly because in these diseases they are the most characteristic and least resemble those of acute diseases, and if a cure is to be effected they cannot be too accurately noted; partly because the patients become so used to their long sufferings that they pay little or no heed to the lesser accessory symptoms, which are often very pregnant with

---

[87] In chronic diseases of females it is specially necessary to pay attention to pregnancy, sterility, sexual desire, accouchements, miscarriages, suckling, and the state of the menstrual discharge. With respect to the last-named more particularly, we should not neglect to ascertain if it recurs at too short intervals, or is delayed beyond the proper time, how many days it lasts, whether its flow is continuous or interrupted, what is its general quantity, how dark is its color, whether there is leucorrhœa before its appearance or after its termination, but especially by what bodily or mental ailments, what sensations and pains, it is preceded, accompanied or followed; if there is leucorrhœa, what is

its nature, what sensations attend its flow, in what quantity it is, and what are the conditions and occasions under which it occurs?

meaning (characteristic)—often very useful in determining the choice of the remedy—and regard them almost as a necessary part of their condition, almost as health, the real feeling of which they have well-nigh forgotten in their sometimes fifteen or twenty years of suffering, and they can scarcely bring themselves to believe that these accessory symptoms, these greater or lesser deviations from the healthy state, can have any connection with their principal malady.

§ 96.

Besides this, patients themselves differ so much in their dispositions, that some, especially the so-called hypochondriacs and other persons of great sensitiveness and impatient of suffering, portray their symptoms in too vivid colors and, in order to induce the physician to give them relief, describe their ailments in exaggerated expressions.[88]

---

[88] A pure fabrication of symptoms and sufferings will never be met with in hypochondriacs, even in the most impatient of them—a comparison of the sufferings they complain of at various times when the physician gives them nothing at all, or something quite unmedicinal, proves this plainly;—but we must deduct something from their exaggeration, at all events ascribe the strong character of their expressions to their excessive sensibility, in which case this very exaggeration of their expressions when talking of their ailments becomes of itself an important symptom in the list of features of which the portrait of the disease is composed. The case is different with insane persons and rascally feigners of disease.

§ 97.

Other individuals of an opposite character, however, partly from indolence, partly from false modesty, partly from a kind of mildness of disposition or weakness of mind, refrain from mentioning a number of their symptoms, describe them in vague terms, or allege some of them to be of no consequence.

§ 98.

Now, as certainly as we should listen particularly to the patient's description of his sufferings and sensations, and attach credence especially to his own expressions wherewith he endeavors to make us understand his ailments—because in the mouths of his friends and attendants they are usually altered and erroneously stated—so certainly, on the other hand, in all diseases, but especially in the chronic ones, the investigation of the true, complete picture and its peculiarities demands especial circumspection, tact, knowledge of human nature, caution in conducting the inquiry and patience in an eminent degree.

§ 99.

On the whole, the investigation of acute diseases, or of such as have existed but a short time, is much the easiest for the physician, because all the phenomena and deviations from the health that has been but recently lost are still fresh in the memory of the patient and his friends, still continue to be novel and striking. The physician certainly requires to know everything in such cases also; but he has much less to *inquire into;* they are for the most part spontaneously detailed to him.

§ 100.

In investigating the totality of the symptoms of epidemic and sporadic diseases it is quite immaterial whether or not something similar has ever appeared in the world before under the same or any other name. The novelty or peculiarity of a disease of that kind makes no difference either in the mode of examining or of treating it, as the physician must any way regard the pure picture of every prevaling disease as if it were something new and unknown, and investigate it thoroughly for itself, if he desire to practice medicine in a real and radical manner, never substituting conjecture for actual observation, never taking for granted that the case of disease before him is already wholly or partially known, but always carefully examining it in all its phases; and this mode of procedure is all the more requisite in such cases, as a careful examination will show that every prevailing disease is in many respects a phenomenon of a unique character, differing vastly from all previous epidemics, to which certain names have been falsely applied—with the exception of those epidemics resulting from a contagious principle that always remains the same, such as small pox, measles, etc.

§ 101.

It may easily happen that in the first case of an epidemic disease that presents itself to the physician's notice he does not at once obtain a knowledge of its complete picture, as it is only by a close observation of several cases of every such collective disease that he can become conversant with the totality of its signs and symptoms. The carefully observing physician can, however, from the examination of even the first and second patients, often arrive so nearly at a knowledge of the true state as to have in his mind a characteristic portrait of it, and even to succeed in finding a suitable, homœopathically adapted remedy for it.

§ 102.

In the course of writing down the symptoms of several cases of this kind the sketch of the disease picture becomes ever more and more complete, not more spun out and verbose, but more significant (more characteristic), and including more of the peculiarities of this collective disease; on the one hand, the general symptoms (e. g., loss of appetite, sleeplessness, etc) become precisely defined as to their peculiarities; and on the other, the more marked and special symptoms which are peculiar to but few diseases and of rarer occurrence, at least in the same combination, become prominent and constitute what is characteristic of this malady.[89] All those af-

---

[89] The physician who has already, in the first cases, been able to choose a remedy approximating to the homœopathic specific, will, from the subsequent cases, be enabled either to verify the suitableness of the medicine chosen, or to discover a more appropriate, the most appropriate homœopathic remedy.

fected with the disease prevailing at a given time have certainly contracted it from one and the same source and hence are suffering from the *same* disease; but the whole extent of such an epidemic disease and the totality of its symptoms (the knowledge whereof, which is essential for enabling us to choose the most suitable homœopathic remedy for this array of symptoms, is obtained by a complete survey of the morbid picture) cannot be learned from one single patient, but is only to be perfectly deduced (abstracted) and ascertained from the sufferings of several patients of different constitutions.

§ 103.

In the same manner as has here been taught relative to the epidemic diseases, which are generally of an acute character, the miasmatic chronic maladies, which, as I have shown, always remain the same in their essential nature, especially the psora, must be investigated, as to the whole sphere of their symptoms, in a much more minute manner than has ever been done before, for in them also one patient only exhibits a portion of their symptoms, a second, a third, and so on, present some other symptoms, which also are but a (dissevered, as it were) portion of the totality of the symptoms which constitute the entire extent of this malady, so that the whole array of the symptoms belonging to such a miasmatic, chronic disease, and especially to the psora, can only be ascertained from the observation of *very many* single patients affected with such a chronic disease, and without a complete survey and collective picture of these symptoms the medicines capable of curing the whole malady homœopathically (to wit, the antipsorics) cannot be discovered; and these medicines are, at the same time, the true remedies of the several patients suffering from such chronic affections.

§ 104.

When the totality of the symptoms that specially mark and distinguish the case of disease or, in other words, when the picture of the disease, whatever be its kind, is once accurately sketched,[90] the most difficult part of the

---

[90] The old school physician gave himself very little trouble in this matter in his mode of treatment. He would not listen to any minute detail of all the circumstances of his case by the patient; indeed, he frequently cut him short in his relation of his sufferings, in order that he might not be delayed in the rapid writing of his prescription, composed of a variety of ingredients unknown to him in their true effects. No allopathic physician, as has been said, sought to learn all the minute circumstances of the patient's case, *and still less did he make a note in writing of them.* On seeing the patient again several days afterwards, he recollected nothing concerning the few details he had heard at the first visit (having in the meantime seen so many other patients laboring under different affections); he had allowed everything to go in at one ear and out at the other. At subsequent visits he only asked a few general questions, went through the ceremony of feeling the pulse at the wrist, looked at the tongue, and at the same moment wrote another prescription, on equally irrational principles, or ordered the first one to be continued (in considerable quantities several times a day), and, with a graceful bow, he hurried off to the fiftieth or sixtieth patient he had to visit, in this thoughtless way, in the course of

task is accomplished. The physician has then the picture of the disease, especially if it be a chronic one, always before him to giude him in his treatment; he can investigate it in all its parts and can pick out the characteristic symptoms, in order to oppose to these, that is to say, to the whole malady itself, a very similar artificial morbific force, in the shape of a homœopathically chosen medicinal substance, selected from the lists of symptoms of all the medicines whose pure effects have been ascertained. And when, during the treatment, he wishes to ascertain what has been the effect of the medicine, and what change has taken place in the patient's state, at this fresh examination of the patient he only needs to strike out of the list of the symptoms noted down at the first visit those that have become ameliorated, to mark what still remain, and add any new symptoms that may have supervened.

§ 105.

The second point of the business of a true physician relates to *acquiring a knowledge of the instruments intended for the cure of the natural diseases,* investigating

---

that forenoon. The profession which of all others requires actually the most reflection, a conscientious, careful examination of the state of each individual patient and a special treatment founded thereon, was conducted in this manner by persons who called themselves physicians, *rational practitioners.* The result, as might naturally be expected, was almost invariably bad; and yet patients had to go to them for advice, partly because there were none better to be had, partly for fashion's sake.

the pathogenetic power of the medicines, in order, when called on to cure, to be able to select from among them one, from the list of whose symptoms an artificial disease may be constructed, as similar as possible to the totality of the principal symptoms of the natural disease sought to be cured.

§ 106.

The whole pathogenetic effects of the several medicines must be known; that is to say, all the morbid symptoms and alterations in the health that each of them is specially capable of developing in the healthy individual must first have been observed as far as possible before we can hope to be able to find among them, and to select, suitable homœopathic remedies for most of the natural diseases.

§ 107.

If, in order to ascertain this, medicines be given to *sick* persons, only, even though they be administered singly and alone, then little or nothing precise is seen of their true effects, as those peculiar alterations of the health to be expected from the medicine are mixed up with the symptoms of the disease and can seldom be distinctly observed.

§ 108.

There is, therefore, no other possible way in which the peculiar effects of medicines on the health of individuals can be accurately ascertained—there is no sure, no more natural way of accomplishing this object, than to administer the several medicines experimentally, in moderate doses, to *healthy* persons, in order to ascertain what changes, symptoms and signs of their influence each individually produces on the health of the body and of the mind; that is to say, what disease elements they are able and tend to produce,[91] since, as has been demonstrated (§§ 24-27), all the curative power of medicines lies in this power they possess of changing the state of man's health, and is revealed by observation of the latter.

§ 109.

I was the first that opened up this path, which I have pursued with a perseverance that could only arise and be kept up by a perfect conviction of the great truth, fraught

---

[91] Not one single physician, as far as I know, during the previous two thousand five hundred years, thought of this so natural, so absolutely necessary and only genuine mode of testing medicines for their pure and peculiar effects in deranging the health of man, in order to learn what morbid state each medicine is capable of curing, except the great and immortal Albrecht von Haller. He alone, besides myself, saw the necessity of this (*vide* the Preface to the *Pharmacopœia Helvet.*, Basil, 1771, fol., p. 12) : Nempe primum in corpore *sano* medela tentanda est, *sine peregrina ulla miscela;* odoreque et sapore ejus exploratis, exigua illius dosis ingerenda et ad omnes, quæ inde contingunt, affectiones, quis pulsus, qui calor, quæ respiratio, quænam excretiones, attendendum. Inde ad ductum phænomenorum, in sano obviorum, transeas ad experimenta in corpore ægroto," etc. But *no one, not a single physician,* attended to or followed up this invaluable hint.

with such blessings to humanity, that it is only by the homœopathic employment of medicines[92] that the certain cure of human maladies is possible.[93]

§ 110.

I saw, moreover, that the morbid lesions which previous authors had observed to result from medicinal substances

---

[92] It is impossible that there can be another true, best method of curing dynamic diseases (*i. e.*, all diseases not strictly surgical) besides homœopathy, just as it is impossible to draw more than one straight line betwixt two given points. He who imagines that there are other modes of curing diseases besides it could not have appreciated homœopathy fundamentally nor practised it with sufficient care, nor could he ever have seen or read cases of properly performed homœopathic cures; nor, on the other hand, could he have discerned the baselessness of all allopathic modes of treating diseases and their bad or even dreadful effects, if, with such lax indifference, he places the only true healing art on an equality with those hurtful methods of treatment, or alleges the latter to be auxiliaries to homœopathy which it could not do without! My true, conscientious followers, the pure homœopathists, with their successful, almost never-failing treatment, might teach these persons better.

[93] The first fruits of these labors, as perfect as they could be at that time, I recorded in the *Fragmenta de viribus medicamentorum positivis, sive in sano corpore humano observatis,* pts. i, ii, Lipsiæ, 8, 1805, ap. J. A. Barth; the more mature fruits in the *Reine Arzneimittellehre,* I Th., dritte Ausg.; II Th., dritte Ausg., 1833; III Th., zweite Ausg., 1825; IV Th., zw. Ausg., 1825; V Th., zw. Ausg., 1826; VI Th., zw. Ausg., 1827 [English translation, *Materia Medica Pura,* vols. i and ii]; and in the second, third, and fourth parts of *Die chronischen Krankheiten,* 1828, 1830, Dresden bei Arnold [2nd edit., with a fifth part, Düsseldorf bei Schaub, 1835, 1839].

when taken into the stomach of healthy persons, either in large doses given by mistake or in order to produce death in themselves or others, or under other circumstances, accorded very much with my own observations when experimenting with the same substances on myself and other healthy individuals. These authors give details of what occurred as histories of poisoning and as proofs of the pernicious effects of these powerful substances, chiefly in order to warn others from their use; partly also for the sake of exalting their own skill, when, under the use of the remedies they employed to combat these dangerous accidents, health gradually returned; but partly also, when the persons so affected died under their treatment, in order to seek their own justification in the dangerous character of these substances, which they then termed poisons. None of these observers ever dreamed that the symptoms they recorded merely as proofs of the noxious and poisonous character of these substances were sure revelations of the power of these drugs to extinguish curatively similar symptoms occurring in natural diseases, that these their pathogenetic phenomena were intimations of their homœopathic curative action, and that the only possible way to ascertain their medicinal powers is to observe those changes of health medicines are capable of producing in the healthy organism; for the pure, peculiar powers of medicines available for the cure of disease are to be learned neither by any ingenious *a priori* speculations, nor by the smell, taste or appearance of the drugs, nor by their chemical analysis, nor yet by the employment of several of them at one time in a mixture (prescription) in diseases; it was never suspected that these histories of

13

medicinal diseases would one day furnish the first rudiments of the true, pure materia medica, which from the earliest times until now has consisted solely of false conjectures and fictions of the imagination—that is to say, did not exist at all.[94]

§ 111.

The agreement of my observations on the pure effects of medicines with these older ones—although they were recorded without reference to any therapeutic object—and the very concordance of these accounts with others of the same kind by different authors must easily convince us that medicinal substances act in the morbid changes they produce in the healthy human body *according to fixed, eternal laws of nature,* and by virtue of these are enabled to produce *certain, reliable disease symptoms each according to its own peculiar character.*

§ 112.

In those older prescriptions of the often dangerous effects of medicines ingested in excessively large doses we notice certain states that were produced, not at the commencement, but towards the termination of these sad events, and which were of an exactly opposite nature to

---

[94] See what I have said on this subject in the "Examination of the Sources of the Ordinary Materia Medica," prefixed to the third part of my *Reine Arzneimittellehre* [translated in the *Materia Medica Pura,* vol. ii].

those that first appeared. These symptoms, the very reverse of the *primary action* (§ 63) or proper action of the medicines on the vital force, are the reaction of the vital force of the organism, its *secondary action* (§§ 62-67), of which, however, there is seldom or hardly ever the least trace from experiments with moderate doses on healthy bodies, and from small doses none whatever. In the homœopathic curative operation the living organism reacts from these only so much as is requisite to raise the health again to the normal healthy state (§ 67).

§ 113.

The only exceptions to this are the narcotic medicines. As they, in their primary action, take away sometimes the sensibility and sensation, sometimes the irritability, it frequently happens that in their *secondary action,* even from moderate experimental doses on healthy bodies, an increased sensibility (and a greater irritability) is observable.

§ 114.

With the exception of these narcotic substances, in experiments with moderate doses of medicine on healthy bodies, we observe only their primary action, *i. e.,* those symptoms wherewith the medicine deranges the health of the human being and develops in him a morbid state of longer or shorter duration.

§ 115.

Among these symptoms, there occur in the case of some medicines not a few which are partially, or under certain conditions, directly opposite to other symptoms that have previously or subsequently appeared, but which are not therefore to be regarded as actual *secondary action* or the mere reaction of the vital force, but which only represent the alternating state of the various paroxysms of the primary action; they are termed *alternating actions*.

§ 116.

Some symptoms are produced by the medicines more frequently—that is to say, in many individuals, others more rarely or in few persons, some only in very few healthy bodies.

§ 117.

To the latter category belong the so-called *idiosyncrasies*, by which are meant peculiar corporeal constitutions which, although otherwise healthy, possess a disposition to be brought into a more or less morbid state by certain things which *seem* to produce no impression and no change in many other individuals.[95] But this

---

[95] Some few persons are apt to faint from the smell of roses and to fall into many other morbid, and sometimes dangerous states from partaking of mussels, crabs or the roe of the barbel, from touching the leaves of some kinds of sumach, etc.

inability to make an impression on every one is only *apparent*. For as two things are required for the production of these as well as all other morbid alterations in the health of man—to wit, the inherent power of the influencing substance, and the capability of the vital force that animates the organism to be influenced by it—the obvious derangements of health in the so-called idiosyncrasies cannot be laid to the account of these peculiar constitutions alone, but they must also be ascribed to these things that produce them, in which must lie the power of making the same impressions on all human bodies, yet in such a manner that but a small number of healthy constitutions have a tendency to allow themselves to be brought into such an obvious morbid condition by them. That these agents do actually make this impression on every healthy body is shown by this, that when employed as remedies they render effectual homœopathic service[96] to *all* sick persons for morbid symptoms similar to those they seem to be only capable of producing in so-called idiosyncratic individuals.

§ 118.

Every medicine exhibits peculiar actions on the human frame, which are not produced in exactly the

---

[96] Thus the Princess Maria Porphyroghnita restored her brother, the Emperor Alexius, who suffered from faintings, by sprinkling him with rose water in the presence of his aunt Eudoxia (*Hist. byz. Alexias,* lib. xv, p. 503, ed. Posser) ; and Horstius (*Oper.,* iii, p. 59) saw great benefit from rose vinegar in cases of syncope.

same manner by any other medicinal substance of a different kind.[97]

§ 119.

As certainly as every species of plant differs in its external form, mode of life and growth, in its taste and smell from every other species and genus of plant, as certainly as every mineral and salt differs from all others, in its external as well as its internal physical and chemical properties (which alone should have sufficed to prevent any confounding of one with another), so certainly do they all differ and diverge among themselves in their pathogenetic—consequently also in their therapeutic— effects.[98] Each of these substances produces alterations

---

[97] This fact was also perceived by the estimable A. v. Haller, who says (Preface to his *Hist. stirp. helv.*): "Latet immensa virium diversitas in iis ipsis plantis, quarum facies externas dudum novimus, animas quasi et quodcunque cælestius habent, nondum perspeximus."

[98] Anyone who has a thorough knowledge of, and can appreciate the remarkable difference of, effects on the health of man of every single substance from those of every other, will readily perceive that among them there can be, in a medical point of view, no equivalent remedies whatever, no *surrogates*. Only those who do *not* know the pure, positive effects of the different medicines can be so foolish as to try to persuade us that one can serve in the stead of the other, and can in the same disease prove just as serviceable as the other. Thus do ignorant children confound the most essentially different things, because they scarcely know their external appearances, far less their real value, their true importance and their very dissimilar inherent properties.

in the health of human beings in a peculiar, different, yet determinate manner, so as to preclude the possibility of confounding one with another.[99]

---

[99] If this be pure truth, as it undoubtedly is, then no physician who would not be regarded as devoid of reason, and who would not act contrary to the dictates of his conscience, the sole arbiter of real worth, can employ in the treatment of diseases any medicinal substance but one with whose real significance he is thoroughly and perfectly conversant, *i. e.*, whose positive action on the health of healthy individuals he has so accurately tested that he knows for certain that it is capable of producing a very similar morbid state, more similar than any other medicine with which he is perfectly acquainted, to that presented by the case of disease he intends to cure by means of it; for, as has been shown above, neither man, nor mighty Nature herself, can effect a perfect, rapid and permanent cure otherwise than with a homœopathic remedy. Henceforth no true physician can abstain from making such experiment, in order to obtain this most necessary and only knowledge of the medicines that are essential to cure, this knowledge which has hitherto been neglected by the physicians in all ages. In all former ages—posterity will scarcely believe it—physicians have hitherto contented themselves with blindly prescribing for diseases medicines whose value was unknown, and which had *never been tested* relative to their highly important, very various, pure dynamic action on the health of man; and, moreover, they mingled several of these unknown medicines that differed so vastly among each other in one formula, and left it to *chance* to determine what effect should thereby be produced on the patient. This is just as if a madman should force his way into the workshop of an artisan, seize upon *handfuls of very different tools, with the uses of all of which he is quite unacquainted,* in order, as he imagines, to work at the objects of art he sees around him. I need hardly remark that these would be destroyed, I may say utterly ruined, by his senseless operations.

§ 120.

Therefore medicines, on which depend man's life and death, disease and health, must be thoroughly and most carefully distinguished from one another, and for this purpose tested by careful, pure experiments on the healthy body for the purpose of ascertaining their powers and real effects, in order to obtain an accurate knowledge of them, and to enable us to avoid any mistake in their employment in diseases, for it is only by correct selection of them that the greatest of all earthly blessings, the health of the body and of the mind, can be rapidly and permanently restored.

§ 121.

In proving medicines to ascertain their effects on the healthy body, it must be borne in mind that the strong, heroic substances, as they are termed, are liable even in small doses to produce changes in the health even of robust persons. Those of milder power must be given for these experiments in more considerable quantities; in order to observe the action of the very weakest, however, the subjects of experiment should be persons free from disease, and who are delicate, irritable and sensitive.

§ 122.

In these experiments—on which depends the exactitude of the whole medical art, and the weal of all future generations of mankind—no other medicines should be employed except such as are perfectly well known, and of whose purity, genuineness and energy we are thoroughly assured.

§ 123.

Each of these medicines must be taken in a perfectly simple, unadulterated form; the indigenous plants in the form of freshly expressed juice, mixed with a little alcohol to prevent it spoiling; exotic vegetable substances, however, in the form of powder, or tincture prepared with alcohol when they were in the fresh state, and afterwards mingled with a certain proportion of water; salts and gums, however, should be dissolved in water just before being taken. If the plant can only be procured in its dry state, and if its powers are naturally weak, in that case there may be used for the experiment an infusion of it, made by cutting the herb into small pieces and pouring boiling water on it, so as to extract its medicinal parts; immediately after its preparation it must be swallowed whilst still warm, as all expressed vegetable juices and all aqueous infusions of herbs, without the addition of spirit, pass rapidly into fermentation and decomposition, whereby all their medicinal properties are lost.

§ 124.

For these experiments every medicinal substance must be employed quite alone and perfectly pure, without the admixture of any foreign substance, and without taking anything else of a medicinal nature the same day, nor yet on the subsequent days, nor during all the time we wish to observe the effects of the medicine.

§ 125.

During all the time the experiment lasts the diet must be strictly regulated; it should be as much as possible destitute of spices, of a purely nutritious and simple character, green vegetables,[100] roots and all salads and herb soups (which, even when most carefully prepared, possess some disturbing medicinal qualities) should be avoided. The drinks are to be those usually partaken of, as little stimulating as possible.[101]

§ 126.

The person who is proving the medicine must be pre-eminently trustworthy and conscientious and during the whole time of the experiment avoid all over-exertion of mind and body, all sorts of dissipation and disturbing passions; he should have no urgent business to distract

---

[100] Young green peas, green French beans, boiled potatoes and in all cases carrots are allowable, as the least medicinal vegetables.

[101] The subject of experiment must either be not in the habit of taking pure wine, brandy, coffee or tea, or he must have totally abstained for a considerable time previously from the use of these injurious beverages, some of which are stimulating, others medicinal.

his attention; he must devote himself to careful self-observation and not be disturbed whilst so engaged; his body must be in what is for him a good state of health, and he must possess a sufficient amount of intelligence to be able to express and describe his sensations in accurate terms.

§ 127.

The medicines must be tested on both males and females, in order also to reveal the alterations of the health they produce in the sexual sphere.

§ 128.

The most recent observations have shown that medicinal substances, when taken in their crude state by the experimenter for the purpose of testing their peculiar effects, do not exhibit nearly the full amount of the powers that lie hidden in them which they do when they are taken for the same object in high dilutions potentized by proper trituration and succussion, by which simple operations the powers which in their crude state lay hidden, and as it were dormant, are developed and roused into activity to an incredible extent. In this manner we now find it best to investigate the medicinal powers even of such substances as are deemed weak, and the plan we adopt is to give to the experimenter, on an empty stomach, daily from four to six very small globules of the thirtieth potency of such a substance, moistened with a little water or dissolved in more or less water and thoroughly mixed, and let him continue this for several days.

§ 129.

If the effects that result from such a dose are but slight, a few more globules may be taken daily, until they become more distinct and stronger and the alterations of the health more conspicuous; for not all persons are affected by a medicine in an equally great degree; on the contrary, there is a vast variety in this respect, so that sometimes an apparently weak individual may be scarcely at all affected by moderate doses of a medicine known to be of a powerful character, whilst he is strongly enough acted on by others of a much weaker kind. And, on the other hand, there are very robust persons who experience very considerable morbid symptoms from an apparently mild medicine and only slight symptoms from stronger drugs. Now, as this cannot be known beforehand, it is advisable to commence in every instance with a small dose of the drug and, where suitable and requisite, to increase the dose more and more from day to day.

§ 130.

If, at the very commencement, the first dose administered shall have been sufficiently strong, this advantage is gained, that the experimenter learns the order of succession of the symptoms and can note down accurately the period at which each occurs, which is very useful in leading to a knowledge of the genius of the medicine, for then the order of the primary actions, as also that of the alternating actions, is observed in the most unambiguous manner. A very moderate dose even, often suffices for the experiment, provided only the experimenter is endowed with sufficiently delicate sensitiveness, and is very attentive to his sensations. The duration of the action of a drug can only be ascertained by a comparison of several experiments.

§ 131.

If, however, in order to ascertain anything at all, the same medicine must be given to the same person to test for several successive days in ever-increasing doses, we thereby learn, no doubt, the various morbid states this medicine is capable of producing in a general manner, but we do not ascertain their order of succession; and the subsequent dose often removes, curatively, some one or other of the symptoms caused by the previous dose, or develops in its stead an opposite state; such symptoms should be inclosed in brackets, to mark their ambiguity, until subsequent purer experiments show whether they are the reaction of the organism and secondary action or an alternating action of this medicine.

§ 132.

But when the object is, without reference to the sequential order of the phenomena and the duration of the action of the drug, only to ascertain the symptoms themselves, especially those of a weak medicinal substance, in that case the preferable course to pursue is to give it for several successive days, increasing the dose every day. In this manner the action of an unknown medicine, even of the mildest nature, will be revealed, especially if tested on sensitive persons.

§ 133.

On experiencing any particular sensation from the medicine, it is useful, indeed necessary, in order to determine the exact character of the symptom, to assume various positions while it lasts, and to observe whether, by moving the part affected, by walking in the room or the open air, by standing, sitting or lying the symptom is increased, diminished or removed, and whether it returns on again assuming the position in which it was first observed,—whether it is altered by eating or drinking, or by any other condition, or by speaking, coughing, sneezing or any other action of the body, and at the same time to note at what time of the day or night it usually occurs in the most marked manner, whereby what is peculiar to and characteristic of each symptom will become apparent.

§ 134.

All external influences, and more especially medicines, possess the property of producing in the health of the living organism a particular kind of alteration peculiar to themselves; but all the symptoms peculiar to a medicine do not appear in one person, nor all at once, nor in the same experiment, but some occur in one person chiefly at one time, others again during a second or third trial; in another person some other symptoms appear, but in such a manner that probably some of the phenomena are observed in the fourth, eighth or tenth person which had already appeared in the second, sixth or ninth person, and so forth; moreover, they may not recur at the same hour.

§ 135.

The whole of the elements of disease a medicine is capable of producing can only be brought to anything like completeness by numerous observations on suitable persons of both sexes and of various constitutions. We can only be assured that a medicine has been thoroughly proved in regard to the morbid states it can produce— that is to say, in regard to its pure powers of altering the health of man—when subsequent experimenters can notice little of a novel character from its action, and almost always only the same symptoms as had been already observed by others.

§ 136.

Although, as has been said, a medicine, on being proved on healthy subjects cannot develop in one person all the alterations of health it is capable of causing, but can only do this when given to many different individuals, varying in their corporeal and mental constitution, yet the tendency to excite all these symptoms in every human being exists in it (§ 117), according to an eternal and immutable law of nature, by virtue of which all its effects, even those that are but rarely developed in the healthy person, are brought into operation in the case of every individual if administered to him when he is in a morbid state presenting similar symptoms; it then, even in the smallest dose, being homœopathically selected, silently produces in the patient an artificial state closely resembling the natural disease, which rapidly and permanently (homœopathically) frees and cures him of his original malady.

§ 137.

The more moderate, within certain limits, the doses of the medicine used for such experiments are—provided we endeavor to facilitate the observation by the selection of a person who is a lover of truth, temperate in all respects, of delicate feelings and who can direct the most minute attention to his sensations—so much the more distinctly are the primary effects developed, and only these, which are most worth knowing, occur without any admixture of secondary effects or reactions of the vital force. When, however, excessively large doses are used there occur at the same time not only a number of secondary effects among the symptoms, but the primary effects also come on in such hurried confusion and with such impetuosity that nothing can be accurately observed; let alone the danger attending them, which no one who has any

regard for his fellow-creatures, and who looks on the
meanest of mankind as his brother, will deem an indifferent manner.

§ 138.

All the sufferings, accidents and changes of the health
of the experimenter during the action of a medicine (provided the above conditions [§§ 124-127] essential to a
good and pure experiment are complied with) are solely
derived from this medicine, and must be regarded and
registered as belonging peculiarly to this medicine, as
symptoms of this medicine, even though the experimenter
had observed, *a considerable time previously,* the spontaneous occurrence of similar phenomena in himself.
The reappearance of these during the trial of the medicine only shows that this individual is by virtue of his
peculiar constitution, particularly disposed to have such
symptoms excited in him. In this case they are the
effect of the medicine; the symptoms do not arise spontaneously while the medicine that has been taken is
exercising an influence over the health of the whole
system, but are produced by the medicine.

§ 139.

When the physician does not make the trial of the
medicine on himself, but gives it to another person, the
latter must note down distinctly the sensations, sufferings, accidents and changes of health he experiences at

the time of their occurrence, mentioning the time after the ingestion of the drug when each symptom arose and, if it lasts long, the period of its duration. The physician looks over the report in the presence of the experimenter immediately after the experiment is concluded, or if the trial lasts several days he does this every day, in order, whilst everything is still fresh in his memory, to question him about the exact nature of every one of these circumstances, and to write down the more precise details so elicited, or to make such alterations as the experimenter may suggest.[102]

§ 140.

If the person cannot write, the physician must be informed by him every day of what has occurred to him, and how it took place. What is noted down as authentic information on this point, however, must be chiefly the voluntary narration of the person who makes the experiment, nothing conjectural and as little as possible derived from answers to leading questions should be admitted; everything must be ascertained with the same caution as I have counselled above (§§ 84-99) for the investigation of the phenomena and for tracing the picture of natural diseases.

---

[102] He who makes known to the medical world the results of such experiments becomes thereby responsible for the trust-and justly so, as the weal of suffering humanity is here at stake. worthiness of the person experimented on and his statements,

§ 141.

But the best provings of the pure effects of simple medicines in altering the human health, and of the artificial diseases and symptoms they are capable of developing in the healthy individual, are those which the healthy, unprejudiced and sensitive *physician institutes on himself* with all the caution and care here enjoined. He knows with the greatest certainty the things he has experienced in his own person.[103]

---

[103] Those trials made by the physician on himself have for him other and inestimable advantages. In the first place, the great truth that the medicinal virtue of all drugs, whereon depends their curative power, lies in the changes of health he has himself undergone from the medicines he has proved, and the morbid states he has himself experienced from them, becomes for him an incontrovertible fact. Again, by such noteworthy observations on himself he will be brought to understand his own sensations, his mode of thinking and his disposition (the foundation of all true wisdom γνῶθι σευτὸν), and he will be also trained to be what every physician ought to be, a good observer. All our observations on others are not nearly so interesting as those made on ourselves. The observer of others must always dread lest the experimenter did not feel exactly what he said, or lest he did not describe his sensations with the most appropriate expressions. He must always remain in doubt whether he has not been deceived, at least to some extent. These obstacles to the knowledge of the truth, which can never be thoroughly surmounted in our investigations of the artificial morbid symptoms that occur in others from the ingestion of medicines, cease entirely when we make the trials on ourselves. He who makes these trials on himself knows for certain what he has felt, and each trial is a new inducement for him to investigate the powers of other medicines. He thus becomes more and more practised

§ 142.

But how some symptoms [104] of the simple medicine employed for a curative purpose can be distinguished amongst the symptoms of the original malady, even in diseases, especially in those of a chronic character that usually remain unaltered, is a subject appertaining to the higher art of judgment, and must be left exclusively to masters in observation.

§ 143.

If we have thus tested on the healthy individual a considerable number of simple medicines and carefully

---

in the art of observing, of such importance to the physician, by continuing to observe himself, the one on whom he can most rely and who will never deceive him; and this he will do all the more zealously as these experiments on himself promise to give him a reliable knowledge of the true value and significance of the instruments of cure that are still to a great degree unknown to our art. Let it not be imagined that such slight indispositions caused by taking medicines for the purpose of proving them can be in the main injurious to the health. Experience shows on the contrary, that the organism of the prover becomes, by these frequent attacks on his health, all the more expert in repelling all external influences inimical to his frame and all artificial and natural morbific noxious agents, and becomes more hardened to resist everything of an injurious character, by means of these moderate experiments on his own person with medicines. His health becomes more unalterable; he becomes more robust, as all experience shows.

[104] Symptoms which, during the whole course of the disease, might have been observed only a long time previously, or never before, consequently new ones, belonging to the medicine.

and faithfully registered all the disease elements and symptoms they are capable of developing as artificial disease-producers, then only have we a true materia medica—a collection of real, pure, reliable [105] modes of action of simple medicinal substances, a volume of the book of nature, wherein is recorded a considerable array of the peculiar changes of the health and symptoms ascertained to belong to each of the powerful medicines, as they were revealed to the attention of the observer, in which the likeness of the (homœopathic) disease elements of many natural diseases to be hereafter cured by them are present, which, in a word, contain artificial morbid states, that furnish for the similar natural morbid states the only true, homœopathic, that is to say, specific, therapeutic instruments for effecting their certain and permanent cure.

§ 144.

From such a materia medica everything that is conjectural, all that is mere assertion or imaginary should be strictly excluded; everything should be the pure language of nature carefully and honestly interrogated.

[105] Latterly it has been the habit to entrust the proving of medicines to unknown persons at a distance, who were paid for their work, and the information so obtained was printed. But by so doing, the work which is of all others the most important, which is to form the basis of the only true healing art, and which demands the greatest moral certainty and trustworthiness, seems to me, I regret to say, to become doubtful and uncertain in its results and to lose all value.

§ 145.

Of a truth it is only by a very considerable store of medicines accurately known in respect of these their pure modes of action in altering the health of man that we can be placed in a position to discover a homœopathic remedy, a suitable artificial (curative) morbific analogue for *each* of the infinitely numerous morbid states in nature, for *every* malady in the world.[106] In the meantime, even now—thanks to the truthful character of the symptoms, and to the abundance of disease elements which every one of the powerful medicinal substances has already shown in its action on the healthy body—but few diseases remain, for which a tolerably suitable homœopathic remedy may not be met with among those now proved as to their pure action,[107] which without much disturbance, restores health in a gentle, sure and permanent manner—*infinitely* more surely and safely than can be effected by all the general

---

[106] At first, about forty years ago, I was the only person who made the proving of the pure powers of medicines the most important of his occupations. Since then I have been assisted in this by some young men, who instituted experiments on themselves, and whose observations I have critically revised. Following these some genuine work of this kind was done by a few others. But what shall we not be able to effect in the way of curing in the whole extent of the infinitely large domain of disease, when numbers of *accurate* and *trustworthy* observers shall have rendered their services in enriching this, the only true materia medica, by careful *experiments on themselves!* The healing art will then come near the mathematical sciences in certainty.

[107] See the second note to § 109.

and special therapeutics of the old allopathic medical art with its unknown composite remedies, which do but alter and aggravate but cannot cure chronic diseases, and rather retard than promote recovery from acute diseases and frequently endanger life.

§ 146.

The third point of the business of a true physician relates to the *judicious employment* of the artificial morbific agents (*medicines*) that have been proved on healthy individuals to ascertain their pure action, *in order to effect the homœopathic cure of natural diseases.*

§ 147.

Whichever of these medicines that have been investigated as to their power of altering man's health we find to contain in the symptoms observed from its use the greatest similarity to the totality of the symptoms of a given natural disease, this medicine will and must be the most suitable, the most certain homœopathic remedy for the disease; in it is found the specific remedy of this case of disease.

§ 148.

The natural disease is never to be considered as a noxious material situated somewhere within the interior or exterior of man (§§ 11-13) but as one produced by an inimical spirit-like (conceptual) agency which, like a kind

of infection (note to § 11) disturbs in its instinctive existence of the spirit-like (conceptual) principle of life within
the organism torturing it as an evil spirit and compelling
it to produce certain ailments and disorders in the regular
course of its life. These are known as symptoms (disease).
If, now, the influence of this inimical agency that not
only caused but strives to continue this disorder, be taken
away as is done when the physician administers an artificial potency, capable of altering the life principle in
the most similar manner (a homœopathic medicine)
which exceeds in energy even in the smallest dose the
similar natural disease (§§ 33, 279), then the influence of
the original noxious morbid agent on the life principle
is lost during the action of this stronger similar artificial
disease. Thence the evil no longer exists for the life
principle—it is destroyed. If, as has been said, the
selected homœopathic remedy is administered properly,
then the acute natural disease which is to be overruled
if recently developed, will disappear unperceptibly in a
few hours.

An older, more chronic disease will yield somewhat
later together with all traces of discomfort, by the use
of several doses of the same more highly potentized remedy or after careful selection [108] of one or another more

---

[108] But this laborious, sometimes very laborious, search for and
selection of the homœopathic remedy most suitable in every respect to each morbid state, is an operation which, notwithstanding all the admirable books for facilitating it, still demands the
study of the original sources themselves, and at the same time
a great amount of circumspection and serious deliberation, which
have their best reward in the consciousness of having faithfully

similar homœopathic medicine. Health, recovery, follow in imperceptible, often rapid transitions. The life

---

discharged our duty. How could his laborious, care-demanding
task, by which alone the best way of curing diseases is rendered
possible, please the gentlemen of the new mongrel sect, who
assume the honorable name of homœopathists, and even seem
to employ medicines in form and appearance homœopathic, but
determined upon by them anyhow (*quidquid in buccam venit*),
and who, when the unsuitable remedy does not immediately give
relief, in place of laying the blame on their unpardonable ignorance and laxity in performing the most important and serious of
all human affairs, ascribe it to homœopathy, which they accuse
of great imperfection (if the truth be told, its imperfection consists in this, that the most suitable homœopathic remedy for
each morbid condition does not spontaneously fly into their
mouths like roasted pigeons, without any trouble on their own
part). They know, however, from frequent practice, how to
make up for the inefficiency of the scarcely half homœopathic
remedy by the employment of allopathic means, that come much
more handy to them, among which one or more dozens of leeches
applied to the affected part, or little harmless venesections to the
extent of eight ounces, and so forth, play an important part; and
should the patient, in spite of all this, recover, they extol their
venesections, leeches, etc., alleging that, had it not been for
these, the patient would not have been pulled through, and they
give us to understand, in no doubtful language, that these operations, derived without much exercise of genius from the pernicious routine of the old school, in reality contributed the best
share towards the cure. But if the patient die under the treatment, as not unfrequently happens, they seek to console the
friends by saying that "they themselves were witnesses that
everything conceivable had been done for the lamented deceased."
Who would do this frivolous and pernicious tribe the honor to
call them, after the name of the very laborious but salutary art,
homœopathic physicians? May the just recompense await them,
that, when taken ill, they may be treated in the same manner!

principle is freed again and capable of resuming the life
of the organism in health as before and strength returns.

§ 149.

Diseases of long standing (and especially such as are
of a complicated character) require for their cure a pro-
portionately longer time. More especially do the chronic
medicinal dyscrasia so often produced by allopathic
bungling along with the natural disease left uncured by
it, require a much longer time for their recovery; often,
indeed, are they incurable, in consequence of the shame-
ful robbery of the patient's strength and juices (venesections, purgatives etc.), on account of long continued
use of large doses of violently acting remedies given on
the basis of empty, false theories for alleged usefulness
in cases of disease appearing similar, also in prescribing
unsuitable mineral baths, etc., the principal feat performed by allopathy in its so-called methods of treatment.

§ 150.

If a patient complain of one or more trivial symptoms,
that have been only observed a short time previously, the
physician should not regard this as a fully developed disease that requires serious medical aid. A slight alteration in the diet and regimen will usually suffice to dispel
such an indisposition.

§ 151.

But if the patient complain of a few violent sufferings, the physician will usually find, on investigation, several other symptoms besides, although of a slighter character, which furnish a complete picture of the disease.

§ 152.

The worse the acute disease is, of so much the more numerous and striking symptoms is it generally composed, but with so much the more certainty may a suitable remedy for it be found, if there be a sufficient number of medicines known, with respect to their positive action, to choose from. Among the lists of symptoms of many medicines it will not be difficult to find one from whose separate disease elements an antitype of curative artificial disease, very like the totality of the symptoms of the natural disease, may be constructed, and such a medicine is the desired remedy.

§ 153.

In this search for a homœopathic specific remedy, that is to say, in this comparison of the collective symptoms of the natural disease with the list of symptoms of known medicines, in order to find among these an artificial mor-bific agent corresponding by similarity to the disease to be cured, the *more striking, singular, uncommon and peculiar* (characteristic) signs and symptoms [109] of the case of disease are chiefly and most solely to be kept in view; for it is *more particularly these that very similar ones in the list of symptoms of the selected medicine must correspond to,* in order to constitute it the most suitable for effecting the cure. The more general and undefined symptoms: loss of appetite, headache, debility, restless sleep, discomfort; and so forth, demand but little attention when of that vague and indefinite character, if they cannot be more accurately described, as symptoms of such a general nature are observed in almost every disease and from almost every drug.

§ 154.

If the antitype constructed from the list of symptoms of the most suitable medicine contain those peculiar, uncommon, singular and distinguishing (characteristic) symptoms, which are to be met with in the disease to be cured in the greatest number and in the greatest similarity, *this* medicine is the most appropriate homœopathic specific remedy for *this* morbid state; the disease, if it be not one of very long standing, will generally be removed and extinguished by the first dose of it, without any considerable disturbance.

---

[109] Dr. von Bönninghausen, by the publication of the characteristic symptoms of homœopathic medicines and his Repertory has rendered a great service to Homœopathy as well as Dr. J. H. G. Jahr in his hand-book of principal symptoms.

§ 155.

I say *without any considerable disturbance.* For in the employment of this most appropriate homœopathic remedy it is only the symptoms of the medicine that correspond to the symptoms of the disease that are called into play, the former occupying the place of the latter (weaker) in the organism, *i. e.,* in the sensations of the life principle, and thereby annihilating them by over-powering them; but the other symptoms of the homœo-pathic medicine, which are often very numerous, being in no way applicable to the case of disease in question, are not called into play at all. The patient, growing hourly better, feels almost nothing of them at all, because the excessively minute dose requisite for homœopathic use is much too weak to produce the other symptoms of the medicine that are not homœopathic to the case, in those parts of the body that are free from disease and consequently can allow only the homœopathic symptoms to act on the parts of the organism that are already most irritated and excited by the similar symptoms of the disease, in order that the sick life principle may react only to a similar but stronger medicinal disease, whereby the original malady is extinguished.

§ 156.

There is, however, almost no homœopathic medicine, be it ever so suitably chosen, that, especially if it should be given in an insufficiently minute dose, will not pro-duce, in very irritable and sensitive patients, at least one trifling, unusual disturbance, some slight new symptom whilst its action lasts; for it is next to impossible that medicine and disease should cover one another symptomatically as exactly as two triangles with equal sides and equal angles. But this (in ordinary circumstances) unimportant difference will be easily done away with by the potential activity (energy) of the living organism, and is not perceptible by patients not excessively delicate; the restoration goes forward, notwithstanding, to the goal of perfect recovery, if it be not prevented by the action of heterogeneous medicinal influences upon the patient, by errors of regimen or by excitement of the passions.

§ 157.

But though it is certain that a homœopathically selected remedy does, by reason of its appropriateness and the minuteness of the dose, gently remove and annihilate the acute disease analogous to it, without manifesting its other unhomœopathic symptoms, that is to say, without the production of new, serious disturbances, yet it usually, immediately after ingestion—for the first hour, or for a few hours—causes a kind of slight aggravation when the dose has not been sufficiently small and (where the dose has been somewhat too large, however, for a considerable number of hours), which has so much resemblance to the original disease that it seems to the patient to be an aggravation of his own disease. But it is, in reality, nothing more than an extremely similar *medicinal disease,* somewhat exceeding in strength the original affection.

§ 158.

This slight *homœopathic* aggravation during the first hours—a very good prognostic that the acute disease will most probably yield to the first dose—is quite as it ought to be, as the medicinal disease must naturally be somewhat stronger than the malady to be cured if it is to overpower and extinguish the latter, just as a natural disease can remove and annihilate another one similar to it only when it is stronger than the latter (§§ 43-48).

§ 159.

The smaller the dose of the homœopathic remedy is in the treatment of acute diseases so much the slighter and shorter is this apparent increase of the disease during the first hours.

§ 160.

But as the dose of a homœopathic remedy can scarcely ever be made so small that it shall not be able to relieve, overpower, indeed completely cure and annihilate the uncomplicated natural disease of not long standing that is analogous to it (§ 249, note), we can understand why a dose of an appropriate homœopathic medicine, not the very smallest possible, does always, during the first hour after its ingestion, produce a perceptible homœopathic aggravation of this kind.[110]

---

[110] This exaltation of the medicinal symptoms over those disease symptoms analogous to them, which looks like an aggravation, has been observed by other physicians also, when by acci-

§ 161.

When I here limit the so-called homœopathic aggravation, or rather the primary action of the homœopathic medicine that seems to increase somewhat the symptoms of the original disease, to the first or few first hours, this is certainly true with respect to diseases of a more acute character and of recent origin; but where medicines of long action have to combat a malady of considerable or of very long standing, where no such apparent increase of the original disease ought to appear during treatment and it does not so appear if the accurately

---

dent they employed a homœopathic remedy. When a patient suffering from itch complains of an increase of the eruption after sulphur, his physician who knows not the cause of this, consoles him with the assurance that the itch must first come out properly before it can be cured; he knows not, however, that this is a sulphur eruption, that assumes the appearance of an increase of the itch.

"The facial eruption which the *viola tricolor* cured was aggravated by it at the commencement of its action," Leroy tells us (*Heilk. für Mütter*, p. 406), but he knew not that the apparent aggravation was owing to the somewhat too large dose of the remedy, which in this instance was to a certain extent homœopathic. Lysons says (*Med. Transact.*, vol. ii, London, 1772), "The bark of the elm cures most certainly those skin diseases which it increases at the beginning of its action." Had he not given the bark in the monstrous doses usual in the allopathic system, but in the quite small doses requisite when the medicine shows similarity of symptoms, that is to say, when it is used homœopathically, he would have effected a cure without, or almost without, seeing this apparent increase of the disease (homœopathic aggravation).

REPRODUCTION OF HAHNEMANN'S HANDWRITING, TAKEN FROM
THE MANUSCRIPT OF THE SIXTH EDITION OF THE ORGANON.

15

auf die erste oder ersten Stunden setze, so ist diess allerdings bei den mehr acuten, seit Kurzem entstandenen Uebeln der Fall [1]; wo aber Arzneien von langer Wirkungsdauer ein altes und sehr altes Siechthum zu bekämpfen haben, eine Gabe also viele Tage allein fortwirken muss, da sieht man in den ersten 6, 8, 10 Tagen von Zeit zu Zeit einige solcher Erstwirkungen der Arznei, einige solche anscheinende Symptomen-Erhöhungen des ursprünglichen Uebels (von einer oder etlichen Stunden Dauer) hervorkommen, während in den Zwischenstunden Besserung des Ganzen sichtbar wird. Nach Verfluss dieser wenigen Tage erfolgt dann die Besserung von solchen Erstwirkungen der Arznei fast ungetrübt noch mehre Tage hindurch.

§. - 162.

Zuweilen trifft sich's bei der noch mässigen Zahl genau nach ihrer wahren, reinen Wirkung gekannter Arzneien, dass nur ein Theil von den Symptomen der zu heilenden Krankheit in der Symptomenreihe der noch am besten passenden Arznei angetroffen wird, folglich

---

1) Die Wirkung derjenigen Arzneien, denen an sich auch die längste Wirkungsdauer eigen ist, in acuten Krankheiten schnell abläuft, am schnellsten in den acutesten — so lang dauernd ist sie doch in (aus Psora entstandnen) chronischen Krankheiten, und daher kommt es, dass die antipsorischen Arzneien oft keine solche homöopathische Verschlimmerung in den ersten Stunden, wohl aber später und in verschiednen Stunden der ersten 8, 10 Tage merken lassen.

O

chosen medicine was given in proper small, gradually higher doses, each somewhat modified with renewed dynamization (§ 247). Such increase of the original symptoms of a chronic disease can appear only at the end of treatment when the cure is almost or quite finished.

§ 162.

It sometimes happens, *owing to the moderate number of medicines yet known with respect to their true, pure* action, that but a *portion* of the symptoms of the disease under treatment is to be met with in the list of symptoms of the most appropriate medicine, consequently this imperfect medicinal morbific agent must be employed for lack of a more perfect one.

§ 163.

In this case we cannot indeed expect from this medicine a complete, undisturbed cure; for during its use some symptoms appear which were not previously observable in the disease, accessory symptoms of the not perfectly appropriate remedy. This does by no means prevent a considerable part of the disease (the symptoms of the disease that resemble those of the medicine) from being eradicated by this medicine thereby establishing a fair commencement of the cure, but still this does not take place without those accessory symptoms, which are, however, always moderate when the dose of the medicine is sufficiently minute.

§ 164.

The small number of homœopathic symptoms present in the best selected medicines is no obstacle to the cure in cases *where these few medicinal symptoms are chiefly of an uncommon kind and such as are peculiarly distinctive* (characteristic) *of the disease;* the cure takes place under such circumstances without any particular disturbance.

rather
than remedy.

§ 165.

If, however, among the symptoms of the remedy selected, there be none that accurately resemble the distinctive (characteristic), peculiar, uncommon symptoms of the case of disease, and if the remedy correspond to the disease only in the general, vaguely described, indefinite states (nausea, debility, headache, and so forth), and if there be among the known medicines none more homœopathically appropriate, in that case the physician cannot promise himself any immediate favorable result from the employment of this unhomœopathic medicine.

§ 166.

Such a case is, however, *very rare,* owing to the increased number of medicines whose pure effects are now known, and the bad effects resulting from it, when they do occur, are diminished whenever a subsequent medicine, of more accurate resemblance, can be selected.

§ 167.

Thus if there occur, during the use of this imperfectly homœopathic remedy first employed, accessory symptoms of some moment, then, in the case of acute diseases, we do not allow this first dose to exhaust its action, nor leave the patient to the full duration of the action of the remedy, but we investigate afresh the morbid state in its now altered condition, and add the remainder of the original symptoms to those newly developed in tracing a new picture of the disease.

§ 168.   *Trial method*

We shall then be able much more readily to discover, among the known medicines, an analogue to the morbid state before us, a single dose of which, if it do not entirely destroy the disease, will advance it considerably on the way to be cured. And thus we go on, if even this medicine be not quite sufficient to effect the restoration of health, examining again and again the morbid state that still remains, and selecting a homœopathic medicine as suitable as possible for it, until our object, namely, putting the patient in the possession of perfect health, is accomplished.

§ 169.

If, on the first examination of a disease and the first selection of a medicine, we should find that the totality of the symptoms of the disease would not be effectually

covered by the disease elements of a single medicine—
owing to the insufficient number of known medicines—
but that two medicines contend for the preference in
point of appropriateness, one of which is more homœopathically suitable for one part, the other for another
part of the symptoms of the disease, it is not advisable,
after the employment of the more suitable of the two
medicines, to administer the other without fresh examination, and much less to give both together (§ 272, note)
for the medicine that seemed to be the next best would
not, under the change of circumstances that has in the
meantime taken place, be suitable for the rest of the
symptoms that then remain; in which case, consequently,
a more appropriate homœopathic remedy must be
selected in place of the second medicine for the set of
symptoms as they appear on a new inspection.

§ 170.

Hence in this as in every case where a change of the
morbid state has occurred, the remaining set of symptoms now present must be inquired into, and (without
paying any attention to the medicine which at first appeared to be the next in point of suitableness) another
homœopathic medicine, as appropriate as possible to the
new state now before us, must be selected. If it should
so happen, as is not often the case, that the medicine
which at first appeared to be the next best seems still
to be well adapted for the morbid state that remains, so
much the more will it merit our confidence, and deserve
to be employed in preference to another.

§ 171.

In non-venereal chronic diseases, those most commonly, therefore, that arise from psora, we often require, in order to effect a cure, to give several antipsoric remedies in succession, every successive one being homœopathically chosen in consonance with the group of symptoms remaining after completion of the action of the previous remedy.

§ 172.

A similar *difficulty* in the way of the cure occurs *from the symptoms of the disease being too few*—a circumstance that deserves our careful attention, for by its removal almost all the difficulties that can lie in the way of this most perfect of all possible modes of treatment (except that its apparatus of known homœopathic medicines is still incomplete) are removed.

§ 173.

The only diseases that seem to have but few symptoms, and on that account to be less amenable to cure, are those which may be termed *one-sided,* because they display only one or two principal symptoms which obscure almost all the others. They belong chiefly to the class of chronic diseases.

§ 174.

Their principal symptom may be either an internal complaint (*e. g.,* a headache of many years' duration, a diarrhœa of long standing, an ancient cardialgia, etc.), or it may be an affection more of an external kind. Diseases of the latter character are generally distinguished by the name of *local maladies*.

§ 175.

In one-sided diseases of the first kind it is often to be attributed to the medical observer's want of discernment that he does not fully discover the symptoms actually present which would enable him to complete the sketch of the portrait of the disease.

§ 176.

There are, however, still a few diseases, which, after the most careful initial examination (§§ 84-98), present but one or two severe, violent symptoms, while all the others are but indistinctly perceptible.

§ 177.

In order to meet most successfully such a case as *this,* which is of *very rare* occurrence, we are in the first place to select, guided by these few symptoms, the medicine which in our judgment is the most homœopathically indicated.

§ 178.

It will, no doubt, sometimes happen that this medicine, selected in strict observance of the homœopathic law,

furnishes the similar artificial disease suited for the
annihilation of the malady present; and this is much more
likely to happen when these few morbid symptoms are
very striking, decided, uncommon and peculiarly distinctive (characteristic).

§ 179.

More frequently, however, the medicine first chosen in
such a case will be only partially, that is to say not
exactly, suitable, as there was no considerable number of
symptoms to guide to an accurate selection.

§ 180.

In this case the medicine, which has been chosen as
well as was possible, but which, for the reason above
stated, is only imperfectly homœopathic, will, in its
action upon the disease that is only partially analogous
to it—just as in the case mentioned above (§ 162,
et seq.), where the limited number of homœopathic remedies renders the selection imperfect—produce accessory
symptoms, and several phenomena from its own array
of symptoms are mixed up with the patient's state of
health, which are, however, at the same time, symptoms
of the disease itself, although they may have been hitherto never or very rarely perceived; some symptoms
which the patient had never previously experienced appear, or others he had only felt indistinctly become more
pronounced.

§ 181.

Let it not be objected that the accessory phenomena and new symptoms of this disease that now appear should be laid to the account of the medicament just employed. They owe their origin to it [111] certainly, but they are always only symptoms of such a nature as *this* disease was itself capable of producing in *this* organism, and which were summoned forth and induced to make their appearance by the medicine given, owing to its power to cause similar symptoms. In a word, we have to regard the whole collection of symptoms now perceptible as belonging to the disease itself, as the actual existing condition, and to direct our further treatment accordingly.

§ 182.

Thus the imperfect selection of the medicament, which was in this case almost inevitable owing to the too limited number of the symptoms present, serves to complete the display of the symptoms of the disease, and in this way facilitates the discovery of a second, more accurately suitable, homœopathic medicine.

§ 183.

Whenever, therefore, the dose of the first medicine ceases to have a beneficial effect (if the newly developed

---

[111] When they were not caused by an important error in regimen, a violent emotion, or a tumultuous revolution in the organism, such as the occurrence or cessation of the menses, conception, childbirth, and so forth.

symptoms do not, by reason of their gravity, demand more speedy aid—which, however, from the minuteness of the dose of homœopathic medicine, and in very chronic diseases, is excessively rare), a new examination of the disease must be instituted, the *status morbi* as it now is must be noted down, and a second homœopathic remedy selected in accordance with it, which shall exactly suit the present state, and one which shall be all the more appropriate can then be found, as the group of symptoms has become larger and more complete.[112]

§ 184.

In like manner, after each new dose of medicine has exhausted its action, when it is no longer suitable and helpful, the state of the disease that still remains is to be noted anew with respect to its remaining symptoms, and another homœopathic remedy sought for, as suitable as possible for the group of symptoms now observed, and so on until the recovery is complete.

---

[112] In cases where the patient (which, however, happens excessively seldom in chronic, but not infrequently in acute, diseases) feels very ill, although his symptoms are very indistinct, so that this state may be attributed more to the benumbed state of the nerves, which does not permit the patient's pains and sufferings to be distinctly perceived, this torpor of the internal sensibility is removed by opium, and in its secondary action the symptoms of the disease become distinctly apparent.

§ 185.

Among the one-sided diseases an important place is occupied by the so-called *local maladies,* by which term is signified those changes and ailments that appear on the external parts of the body. Till now the idea prevalent in the schools was that these parts were alone morbidly affected, and that the rest of the body did not participate in the disease—a theoretical, absurd doctrine, which has led to the most disastrous medical treatment.

§ 186.

Those so-called local maladies which have been produced a short time previously, solely by an external lesion, still appear at first sight to deserve the name of *local* diseases. But then the lesion must be very trivial, and in that case it would be of no great moment. For in the case of injuries accruing to the body from without, if they be at all severe, the whole living organism sympathizes; there occur fever, etc. The treatment of such diseases is relegated to surgery; but this is right only in so far as the affected parts require mechanical aid, whereby the external obstacles to the cure, which can only be expected to take place by the agency of the vital force, may be removed by mechanical means, *e. g.,* by the reduction of dislocations, by needles and bandages to bring together the lips of wounds, by mechanical pressure to still the flow of blood from open arteries, by the extraction of foreign bodies that have penetrated into the living parts, by making an opening into a cavity of the body in order to remove an irritating substance or to procure the evacuation of effusions or collections of fluids, by bringing into apposition the broken extremities of a fractured bone and retaining them in exact contact by an appropriate bandage, etc. But when in such injuries the whole living organism requires, *as it always does,* active *dynamic* aid to put it in a position to accomplish the work of healing, *e. g.,* when the violent fever resulting from extensive contusions, lacerated muscles, tendons and blood-vessels requires to be removed by medicine given internally, or when the external pain of scalded or burnt parts needs to be homœopathically subdued, then the services of the dynamic physician and his helpful homœopathy come into requisition.

§ 187.

But those affections, alterations and ailments appearing on the external parts that do not arise from any external injury or that have only some slight external wound for their immediate exciting cause, are produced in quite another manner; their source lies in some internal malady. To consider them as mere local affections, and at the same time to treat them only, or almost only, as it were surgically, with topical application or other similar remedies—as the old school have done from the remotest ages—is as absurd as it is pernicious in its results.

§ 188.

These affections were considered to be merely topical, and were therefore called *local* diseases, as if they were maladies exclusively limited to those parts wherein the organism took little or no part, or affections of these particular visible parts of which the rest of the living organism, so to speak, knew nothing.[113]

§ 189.

And yet very little reflection will suffice to convince us that no external malady (not occasioned by some important injury from without) can arise, persist or even grow worse without some internal cause, without the co-operation of the whole organism, which must consequently be in a diseased state. It could not make its appearance at all without the consent of the whole of the rest of the health, and without the participation of the rest of the living whole (of the vital force that pervades all the other sensitive and irritable parts of the organism); indeed, it is impossible to conceive its production without the instrumentality of the whole (deranged) life; so intimately are all parts of the organism connected together to form an indivisible whole in sensations and functions. No eruption on the lips, no whitlow can occur without previous and simultaneous internal ill-health.

§ 190.

All true medical treatment of a disease on the external parts of the body that has occurred from little or no

---

[113] One of the many great and pernicious blunders of the old school.

injury from without must, therefore, be directed against
the whole, must effect the annihilation and cure of the
general malady by means of internal remedies, if it is
wished that the treatment should be judicious, sure, efficacious and radical.

§ 191.

This is confirmed in the most unambiguous manner by
experience, which shows in all cases that every powerful
internal medicine immediately after its ingestion causes
important changes in the general health of such a
patient, and particularly in the affected external parts
(which the ordinary medical school regards as quite
isolated), even in a so-called local disease of the most
external parts of the body, and the change it produces
is most salutary, being the restoration to health of the
entire body, along with the disappearance of the external
affection (without the aid of any external remedy), provided the internal remedy directed towards the whole
state was suitably chosen in a homœopathic sense.

§ 192.

This is best effected when, in the investigation of the
case of disease, along with the exact character of the
local affection, all the changes, sufferings and symptoms
observable in the patient's health, and which may have
been previously noticed when no medicines had been
used, are taken in conjunction to form a complete picture

of the disease before searching among the medicines, whose peculiar pathogenetic effects are known, for a remedy corresponding to the totality of the symptoms, so that the selection may be truly homœopathic.

§ 193.

By means of this medicine, employed only internally the general morbid state of the body is removed along with the local affection, and the latter is cured at the same time as the former, proving that the local affection depended solely on a disease of the rest of the body, and should only be regarded as an inseparable part of the whole, as one of the most considerable and striking symptoms of the whole disease.

§ 194.

It is not useful, either in acute local diseases of recent origin or in local affections that have already existed a long time, to rub in or apply externally to the spot an external remedy, even though it be the specific and, when used internally, salutary by reason of its homœopathicity, even although it should be at the same time administered internally; for the acute topical affections (e. g., inflammations of individual parts, erysipelas, etc.), which have not been caused by external injury of proportionate violence, but by dynamic or internal causes, yield most surely to internal remedies homœopathically adapted to the perceptible state of the health present in the exterior and interior, selected from the general store of proved medicines, and generally without any other aid; but if these diseases do not yield to them completely, and if there still remain in the affected spot and in the whole state, notwithstanding good regimen, a relic of disease which the vital force is not competent to restore to the normal state, then the acute disease was (as not infrequently happens) a product of psora which had hitherto remained latent in the interior, but has now burst forth and is on the point of developing into a palpable chronic disease.

§ 195.

In order to effect a radical cure in such cases, which are by no means rare, after the acute state has pretty well subsided, an appropriate antipsoric treatment (as is taught in my work on *Chronic Diseases*) must then be directed against the symptoms that still remain and the morbid state of health to which the patient was previously subject. In chronic local maladies that are not obviously venereal, the antipsoric internal treatment is, moreover, alone requisite.

§ 196.

It might, indeed, seem as though the cure of such diseases would be hastened by employing the medicinal substance which is known to be truly homœopathic to the totality of the symptoms, not only internally, but also externally, because the action of a medicine applied to the seat of the local affection might effect a more rapid change in it.

16

§ 197.

This treatment, however, is quite inadmissible, not only for the local symptoms arising from the miasm of psora, but also and especially for those originating in the miasm of syphilis or sycosis, for *the simultaneous local application, along with the internal employment, of the remedy in diseases whose chief symptom is a constant local affection,* has this great disadvantage, that, by such a topical application, this chief symptom (local affection) [114] will usually be annihilated sooner than the internal disease, and we shall now be deceived by the semblance of a perfect cure; or at least it will be difficult, and in some cases impossible, to determine, from the premature disappearance of the local symptom, if the general disease is destroyed by the simultaneous employment of the internal medicine.

§ 198.

The *mere topical employment* of medicines, that are powerful for cure when given internally, to the local symptoms of chronic miasmatic diseases is for the same reason quite inadmissible; for if the local affection of the chronic disease be only removed locally and in a one-sided manner, the internal treatment indispensable for the complete restoration of the health remains in dubious obscurity; the chief symptom (the local affection) is

---

[114] Recent itch eruption, chancre, condyloma, as I have indicated in my book on Chronic Diseases.

gone, and there remain only the other, less distinguishable symptoms, which are less constant and less persistent than the local affection, and frequently not sufficiently peculiar and too slightly characteristic to display after that, a picture of the disease in clear and peculiar outlines.

§ 199.

If the remedy perfectly homœopathic to the disease had not yet been discovered [115] at the time when the local symptoms were destroyed by a corrosive or desiccative external remedy or by the knife, then the case becomes much more difficult on account of the too indefinite (uncharacteristic) and inconstant appearance of the remaining symptoms; for what might have contributed most to determine the selection of the most suitable remedy, and its internal employment until the disease should have been completely annihilated, namely, the external principal symptom, has been removed from our observation.

§ 200.

Had it still been present to guide the internal treatment, the homœopathic remedy for the whole disease might have been discovered, and had that been found, the persistence of the local affection during its internal employment would have shown that the cure was not yet

---

[115] As was the case before my time with the remedies for the condylomatous disease (and the antipsoric medicines).

completed; but were it cured on its seat, this would be a convincing proof that the disease was completely eradicated, and the desired recovery from the entire disease was fully accomplished, an inestimable, indispensable advantage to reach a perfect cure.

§ 201.

It is evident that man's vital force, when encumbered with a chronic disease which it is unable to overcome by its own powers instinctively, adopts the plan of developing a local malady on some external part, solely for this object, that by making and keeping in a diseased state this part which is not indispensable to human life, it may thereby silence the internal disease, which otherwise threatens to destroy the vital organs (and to deprive the patient of life), and that it may thereby, so to speak, transfer the internal disease to the vicarious local affection and, as it were, draw it thither. The presence of the local affection thus silences, for a time, the internal disease, though without being able either to cure it or to diminish it materially.[118] The local

---

[118] The issues of the old-school practitioners do something similar; as artificial ulcers on external parts, they silence some internal chronic diseases, but only for a very short time, as long as they cause a painful irritation to which the sick organism is not used, without being able to cure them; but, on the other hand, they weaken and destroy the general health much more than is done by most of the metastases effected by the instinctive vital force.

affection, however, is never anything else than a part of the general disease, but a part of it increased all in one direction by the organic vital force, and transferred to a less dangerous (external) part of the body, in order to allay the internal ailment. But (as has been said) by this local symptom that silences the internal disease, so far from anything being gained by the vital force towards diminishing or curing the whole malady, the internal disease, on the contrary, continues, in spite of it, gradually to increase and Nature is constrained to enlarge and aggravate the local symptom always more and more, in order that it may still suffice as a substitute for the increased internal disease and may still keep it under. Old ulcers on the legs get worse as long as the internal psora is uncured, the chancre enlarges as long as the internal syphilis remains uncured, the fig warts increase and grow while the sycosis is not cured whereby the latter is rendered more and more difficult to cure, just as the general internal disease continues to increase as time goes on.

§ 202.

If the old-school physician should now destroy the local symptom by the topical application of external remedies, under the belief that he thereby cures the whole disease, Nature makes up for its loss by rousing the internal malady and the other symptoms that previously existed in a latent state side by side with the local affection; that is to say, she increases the internal disease. When this occurs it is usual to say, though *incorrectly,* that the local affection has been *driven back* into the system or upon the nerves by the external remedies.

§ 203.

Every external treatment of such local symptoms, the object of which is to remove them from the surface of the body, whilst the internal miasmatic disease is left uncured, as, for instance, driving off the skin the psoric eruption by all sorts of ointments, burning away the chancre by caustics and destroying the condylomata on their seat by the knife, the ligature or the actual cautery; this pernicious external mode of treatment, hitherto so universally practised, has been the most prolific source of all the innumerable named or unnamed chronic maladies under which mankind groans; it is one of the most criminal procedures the medical world can be guilty of, and yet it has hitherto been the one generally adopted, and taught from the professional chairs as the only one.[117]

§ 204.

If we deduct all chronic affections, ailments and diseases that depend on a persistent unhealthy mode of

---

[117] For any medicines that might at the same time be given internally served but to aggravate the malady, as these remedies possessed no specific power of curing the whole disease, but assailed the organism, weakened it and inflicted on it, in addition, other chronic medicinal diseases.

living (§ 77), as also those innumerable medicinal maladies (v. § 74) caused by the irrational, persistent, harassing and pernicious treatment of diseases often only of trivial character by physicians of the old school, most the remainder of chronic diseases result from the development of these three chronic miasms, internal syphilis, internal sycosis, but chiefly and in infinitely greater proportion, internal psora. Each of these infections was already in possession of the whole organism, and had penetrated it in all directions before the appearance of the primary, vicarious local symptom of each of them (in the case of psora the scabious eruption, in syphilis the chancre or the bubo, and in sycosis the condylomata) that prevented their outburst; and these chronic miasmatic diseases, if deprived of their local symptom, are inevitably destined by mighty Nature sooner or later to become developed and to burst forth, and thereby propagate all the nameless misery, the incredible number of chronic diseases which have plagued mankind for hundreds and thousands of years, none of which would so frequently have come into existence had physicians striven in a rational manner to cure radically and to extinguish in the organism these three miasms without employing local remedies for their corresponding external symptoms, relying solely on the proper internal homœopathic remedies for each. (See note to § 282.)

§ 205.

The homœopathic physician never treats one of these primary symptoms of chronic miasms, nor yet one of their secondary affections that result from their further development, by local remedies (neither by those external agents that act dynamically,[118] nor yet by those that act mechanically), but he cures, in cases where the one or the other appears, only the great miasm on which they depend, whereupon its primary, as also its secondary symptoms disappear spontaneously; but as this was not the mode pursued by the old-school practitioners who

---

[118] I cannot therefore advise, for instance, the local extirpation of the so-called cancer of the lips and face (the product of highly developed psora, not infrequently in conjunction with syphilis) by means of the arsenical remedy of Frère Cosme, not only because it is excessively painful and often fails, but more for this reason, because, if this dynamic remedy should indeed succeed in freeing the affected part of the body from the malignant ulcer locally, the basic malady is thereby not diminished in the slightest, the preserving vital force is therefore necessitated to transfer the field of operation of the great internal malady to some more important part (as it does in every case of metastasis), and the consequence is blindness, deafness, insanity, suffocative asthma, dropsy, apoplexy, etc. But this ambiguous local liberation of the part from the malignant ulcer by the topical arsenical remedy only succeeds, after all, in those cases where the ulcer has not yet attained any great size, and when the vital force is still very energetic; but it is just in such a state of things that the complete internal cure of the whole original disease is also still practicable.

The result is the same without previous cure of the inner miasm when cancer of the face or breast is removed by the knife alone and when encysted tumors are enucleated; something worse ensues, or at any rate death is hastened. This has been the case times without number, but the old school still goes blindly on in the same way in every new case, with the same disastrous results.

preceded him in the treatment of the case, the homœopathic physician generally, alas! finds that the primary
symptoms [119] have already been destroyed by them by
means of external remedies, and that he has now to do
more with the secondary ones, *i. e.,* the affections resulting from the breaking forth and development of these
inherent miasms, but especially with the chronic diseases evolved from internal psora, the internal treatment
of which, as far as a single physician can elucidate it by
many years of reflection, observation and experience, I
have endeavored to point out in my work on *Chronic
Diseases,* to which I must refer the reader.

§ 206.

Before commencing the treatment of a chronic disease, it is necessary to make the most careful investigation [120] as to whether the patient has had a venereal

---

[119] Itch eruption, chancre (bubo), condylômata.

[120] In investigations of this nature we must not allow ourselves
to be deceived by the assertions of the patients or their friends,
who frequently assign as the cause of chronic, even of the
severest and most inveterate diseases, either a cold caught (a
thorough wetting, drinking cold water after being heated) many
years ago, or a former fright, a sprain, a vexation (sometimes
even a bewitchment), etc. These causes are much too insignificant to develop a chronic disease *in a healthy body,* to keep it
up for years, and to aggravate it year by year, as is the case
with all chronic diseases from developed psora. Causes of a
much more important character than these remembered noxious
influences must lie at the root of the initiation and progress of
a serious, obstinate disease of long standing; the assigned causes
could only rouse into activity the latent chronic miasm.

infection (or an infection with condylomatous gonorrhœa); for then the treatment must be directed towards
this alone, when only the signs of syphilis (or of the
rarer condylomatous disease) are present, but this disease is very seldom met with alone nowadays. If such
infection has previously occurred, this must also be
borne in mind in the treatment of those cases in which
psora is present, because in them the latter is complicated
with the former, as is always the case when the symptoms are not those of pure syphilis; for when the physician thinks he has a case of old venereal disease before
him, he has always, or almost always, to treat a syphilitic
affection accompanied mostly by (complicated with)
psora for the internal itch dyscrasia (the psora) is far
the *most frequent fundamental cause of chronic diseases*. At times, both miasms may be complicated also
with sycosis in chronically diseased organisms, or, as is
much more frequently the case, psora is the sole fundamental cause of all other chronic maladies, whatever
names they may bear, which are, moreover, so often bungled, increased and disfigured to a monstrous extent by
allopathic unskilfulness.

§ 207.

When the above information has been gained, it still
remains for the homœopathic physician to ascertain what
kinds of allopathic treatment had up to that date been
adopted for the chronic disease, what perturbing medicines had been chiefly and most frequently employed, also
what mineral baths had been used and what effects these

had produced, in order to understand in some measure the degeneration of the disease from its original state, and, where possible, to correct in part these pernicious artificial operations, or to enable him to avoid the employment of medicines that have already been improperly used.

§ 208.

The age of the patient, his mode of living and diet, his occupation, his domestic position, his social relations and so forth must next be taken into consideration, in order to ascertain whether these things have tended to increase his malady, or in how far they may favor or hinder the treatment. In like manner the state of his disposition and mind must be attended to, to learn whether that presents any obstacle to the treatment, or requires to be directed, encouraged or modified.

§ 209.

After this is done, the physician should endeavor in repeated conversations with the patient to trace the picture of his disease as completely as possible, according to the directions given above, in order to be able to elucidate the most striking and peculiar (characteristic) symptoms, in accordance with which he selects the first antipsoric or other remedy having the greatest symptomatic resemblance, for the commencement of the treatment, and so forth.

§ 210.

Of psoric origin are almost all those diseases that I have above termed one-sided, which appear to be more difficult to cure in consequence of this one-sidedness, all their other morbid symptoms disappearing, as it were, before the single, great, prominent symptom. Of this character are what are termed *mental diseases*. They do not, however, constitute a class of disease sharply separated from all others, since in all other so-called corporeal diseases the condition of the disposition and mind is *always* altered;[121] and in all cases of disease we are called on to cure the state of the patient's disposition is to be particularly noted, along with the totality of

---

[121] How often, for instance, do we not meet with a mild, soft disposition in patients who have for years been afflicted with the most painful diseases, so that the physician feels constrained to esteem and compassionate the sufferer! But if he subdue the disease and restore the patient to health—as is frequently done in homœopathic practice—he is often astonished and horrified at the frightful alteration in his disposition. He often witnesses the occurrence of ingratitude, cruelty, refined malice and propensities most disgraceful and degrading to humanity, which were precisely the qualities possessed by the patient before he grew ill.

Those who were patient when well often become obstinate, violent, hasty, or even intolerant and capricious, or impatient or desponding when ill; those formerly chaste and modest often become lascivious and shameless. A clear-headed person not infrequently becomes obtuse of intellect, while one ordinarily weak-minded becomes more prudent and thoughtful; and a man slow to make up his mind sometimes acquires great presence of mind and quickness of resolve, etc.

the symptoms, if we would trace an accurate picture of the disease, in order to be able therefrom to treat it homœopathically with success.

§ 211.

This holds good to such an extent, that the state of the disposition of the patient often chiefly determines the selection of the homœopathic remedy, as being a decidedly characteristic symptom which can least of all remain concealed from the accurately observing physician.

§ 212.

The Creator of therapeutic agents has also had particular regard to this main feature of all diseases, the altered state of the disposition and mind, for there is no powerful medicinal substance in the world which does not very notably alter the state of the disposition and mind in the healthy individual who tests it, and every medicine does so in a different manner.

§ 213.

We shall, therefore, never be able to cure conformably to nature—that is to say, homœopathically—if we do not, in every case of disease, even in such as are acute, observe, along with the other symptoms, those relating to the changes in the state of the mind and disposition, and if we do not select, for the patient's relief, from among the medicines a disease-force which in addition to the similarity of its other symptoms to those of the disease, is also capable of producing a similar state of the disposition and mind.[122]

§ 214.

The instructions I have to give relative to the cure of mental diseases may be confined to a very few remarks, as they are to be cured in the same way as all other diseases, namely by a remedy which shows, by the symptoms it causes in the body and mind of a healthy individual, a power of producing a morbid state as similar as possible to the case of disease before us, and in no other way can they be cured.

§ 215.

Almost all the so-called mental and emotional diseases are nothing more than corporeal diseases in which the symptom of derangement of the mind and disposition peculiar to each of them is increased, whilst the corporeal

---

[122] Thus aconite will seldom or *never* effect either a rapid or permanent cure in a patient of a quiet, calm, equable disposition; and just as little will nux vomica be serviceable where the disposition is mild and phlegmatic, pulsatilla where it is happy, gay and obstinate, or ignatia where it is imperturbable and disposed neither to be frightened nor vexed.

symptoms decline (more or less rapidly), till it at length attains the most striking one-sidedness, almost as though it were a local disease in the invisible subtle organ of the mind or disposition.

§ 216.

The cases are not rare in which a so-called corporeal disease that threatens to be fatal—a suppuration of the lungs, or the deterioration of some other important viscus, or some other disease of acute character, *e. g.*, in childbed, etc.—becomes transformed into insanity, into a kind of melancholia or into mania by a rapid increase of the psychical symptoms that were previously present, whereupon the corporeal symptoms lose all their danger; these latter improve almost to perfect health, or rather they decrease to such a degree that their obscured presence can only be detected by the observation of a physician gifted with perseverance and penetration. In this manner they become transformed into a one-sided and, as it were, a local disease, in which the symptom of the mental disturbance, which was at first but slight, increases so as to be the chief symptom, and in a great measure occupies the place of the other (corporeal) symptoms, whose intensity it subdues in a palliative manner, so that, in short, the affections of the grosser corporeal organs become, as it were, transferred and conducted to the almost spiritual mental and emotional organs, which the anatomist has never yet and never will reach with his scalpel.

§ 217.

In these diseases we must be very careful to make ourselves acquainted with the whole of the phenomena, both those belonging to the corporeal symptoms, and also, and indeed particularly, those appertaining to the accurate apprehension of the precise character of the chief symptom of the peculiar and always predominating state of the mind and disposition, in order to discover, for the purpose of extinguishing the entire disease, among the remedies whose pure effects are known, a homœopathic medicinal pathogenetic force—that is to say, a remedy which in its list of symptoms displays, with the greatest possible similarity, not only the corporeal morbid symptoms present in the case of disease before us, but also especially this mental and emotional state.

§ 218.

To this collection of symptoms belongs in the first place the accurate description of all the phenomena of the previous so-called corporeal disease, before it degenerated into a one-sided increase of the psychical symptom, and became a disease of the mind and disposition. This may be learned from the report of the patient's friends.

§ 219.

A comparison of these previous symptoms of the corporeal disease with the traces of them that still remain, though they have become less perceptible (but which even now sometimes become prominent, when a lucid interval and a transient alleviation of the psychical disease occurs), will serve to prove them to be still present, though obscured.

§ 220.

By adding to this the state of the mind and disposition accurately observed by the patient's friends and by the physician himself, we have thus constructed the complete picture of the disease, for which, in order to effect the homœopathic cure of the disease, a medicine capable of producing strikingly similar symptoms, and especially an analogous disorder of the mind, must be sought for among the antipsoric remedies, if the psychical disease has already lasted some time.

§ 221.

If, however, insanity or mania (caused by fright, vexation, the abuse of spirituous liquors, etc.) has suddenly broken out as an acute disease in the patient's ordinary calm state, although it almost always arises from internal psora, like a flame bursting forth from it, yet when it occurs in this acute manner it should not be immediately treated with antipsorics, but in the first place with remedies indicated for it out of the other class of proved medicaments (*e. g.*, aconite, belladonna, stramonium, hyoscyamus, mercury, etc.) in highly potentized, minute, homœopathic doses, in order to subdue it

17

so far that the psora shall for the time revert to its former latent state, wherein the patient appears as if quite well.

§ 222.

But such a patient, who has recovered from an acute mental or emotional disease by the use of these non-antipsoric medicines, should never be regarded as cured; on the contrary, no time should be lost in attempting to free him completely,[123] by means of a prolonged anti-psoric treatment, from the chronic miasm of the psora, which, it is true, has now become once more latent but is quite ready to break out anew; if this be done, there is no fear of another similar attack, if he attend faith-fully to the diet and regimen prescribed for him.

---

[123] It very rarely happens that a mental or emotional disease of long standing ceases spontaneously (for the internal dyscrasia transfers itself again to the grosser corporeal organs); such are the few cases met with now and then, where a former inmate of a madhouse has been dismissed apparently recovered. Hitherto, moreover, all madhouses have continued to be chokefull, so that the multitude of other insane persons who seek for ad-mission into such institutions could scarcely find room in them unless some of the insane in the house died. *Not one is ever really and permanently cured in them!* A convincing proof, among many others, of the complete nullity of the non-healing art hitherto practised, which has been ridiculously honored by allopathic ostentation with the title of *rational medicine.* How often, on the other hand, has not the true healing art, genuine, pure homœopathy, been able to restore such unfortunate beings to the possession of their mental and corporeal health, and to give them back again to their delighted friends and to the world!

§ 223.

But if the antipsoric treatment be omitted, then we may almost assuredly expect, from a much slighter cause than brought on the first attack of the insanity, the speedy occurrence of a new and more lasting and severe fit, during which the psora usually develops itself completely, and passes into either a periodic or continued mental derangement, which is then more difficult to be cured by antipsorics.

§ 224.

If the mental disease be not quite developed, and if it be still somewhat doubtful whether it really arose from a corporeal affection, or did not rather result from faults of education, bad practices, corrupt morals, neglect of the mind, superstition or ignorance; the mode of deciding this point will be, that if it proceed from one or other of the latter causes it will diminish and be improved by sensible friendly exhortations, consolatory arguments, serious representations and sensible advice; whereas a real moral or mental malady, depending on bodily disease, would be speedily aggravated by such a course, the melancholic would become still more dejected, querulous, inconsolable and reserved, the spiteful maniac would thereby become still more exasperated, and the chattering fool would become manifestly more foolish.[124]

---

[124] It would seem as though the mind, in these cases, felt with uneasiness and grief the truth of these rational representations

§ 225.

There are, however, as has just been stated, certainly a few emotional diseases which have not merely been developed into that form out of corporeal diseases, but which, in an inverse manner, the body being but slightly indisposed, originate and are kept up by emotional causes, such as continued anxiety, worry, vexation, wrongs and the frequent occurrence of great fear and fright. This kind of emotional diseases in time destroys the corporeal health, often to a great degree.

§ 226.

It is only such emotional diseases as these, which were first engendered and subsequently kept up by the mind itself, that, *while they are yet recent and before they have made very great inroads on the corporeal state,* may, by means of psychical remedies, such as a display of confidence, friendly exhortations, sensible advice, and often by a well-disguised deception, be rapidly changed into a healthy state of the mind (and with appropriate diet and regimen, seemingly into a healthy state of the body also).

---

and acted upon the body as if it wished to restore the lost harmony, but that the body, by means of its disease, reacted upon the organs of the mind and disposition and put them in still greater disorder by a fresh transference of its sufferings on to them.

§ 227.

But the fundamental cause in these cases also is a psoric miasm, which was only not yet quite near its full development, and for security's sake, the seemingly cured patient should be subjected to a radical antipsoric treatment, in order that he may not again as might easily occur, fall into a similar state of mental disease.

§ 228.

In mental and emotional diseases resulting from corporeal maladies, which can only be cured by homœopathic antipsoric medicine conjoined with carefully regulated mode of life, an appropriate psychical behavior towards the patient on the part of those about him and of the physician must be scrupulously observed, by way of an auxiliary mental regimen. To furious mania we must oppose calm intrepidity and cool, firm resolution—to doleful, querulous lamentation, a mute display of commiseration in looks and gestures—to senseless chattering, a silence not wholly inattentive—to disgusting and abominable conduct and to conversation of a similar character, total inattention. We must merely endeavor to prevent the destruction and injury of surrounding objects, *without reproaching the patient for his acts, and* everything must be arranged in such a way that the necessity for any corporeal punishments and tortures [125] whatever may be avoided. This is so much the

---

[125] It is impossible not to marvel at the hard-heartedness and indiscretion of the medical men in many establishments for

more easily effected, because in the administration of the medicine—the only circumstance in which the employment of coercion could be justified—in the homœopathic system the small doses of the appropriate medicine *never* offend the taste, and may consequently be given to the patient without his knowledge in his drink, so that all compulsion is unnecessary.

§ 229.

On the other hand, contradiction, eager explanations, rude corrections and invectives, as also weak, timorous yielding, are quite out of place with such patients; they are equally pernicious modes of treating mental and emotional maladies. But such patients are most of all exasperated and their complaint aggravated by contumely, fraud, and deceptions that they can detect. *The*

---

patients of this kind, who, without attempting to discover the true and only efficacious mode of curing such diseases, which is by homœopathic *medicinal* (antipsoric) means, content themselves with torturing these most pitiable of all human beings with the most violent blows and other painful torments. By this unconscientious and revolting procedure they debase themselves beneath the level of the turnkeys in a house of correction, for the latter inflict such chastisements as the duty devolving on their office, and on criminals only, whilst the former appear, from a humiliating consciousness of their uselessness as physicians, only to vent their spite at the supposed incurability of mental diseases in harshness towards the pitiable, innocent sufferers, for they are too ignorant to be of any use and too indolent to adopt a judicious mode of treatment.

physician and keeper must always pretend to believe them to be possessed of reason.

All kinds of external disturbing influences on their senses and disposition should be if possible removed; there are no amusements for their clouded spirit, no salutary distractions, no means of instruction, no soothing effects from conversation, books or other things for the soul that pines or frets in the chains of the diseased body, no invigoration for it, but the cure; it is only when the bodily health is changed for the better that tranquillity and comfort again beam upon their mind.[126]

§ 230.

If the antipsoric remedies selected for each particular case of mental or emotional disease (there are incredibly numerous varieties of them) be quite homœopathically suited for the faithfully traced picture of the morbid state, which, if there be a sufficient number of this kind of medicines known in respect of their pure effects, is ascertained by an indefatigable search for the most appropriate homœopathic remedy all the more easily, as the emotional and mental state, constituting the principal symptom of such a patient, is so unmistakably perceptible,—then the most striking improvement in no very long time, which could not be brought about by physicking the patient to death with the largest oft-

---

[126] The treatment of the violent insane maniac and melancholic can take place only in an institution specially arranged for their treatment but not within the family circle of the patient.

repeated doses of all other unsuitable (allopathic) medicines. Indeed, I can confidently assert, from great experience, that the vast superiority of the homœopathic system over all other conceivable methods of the treatment is nowhere displayed in a more triumphant light than in mental and emotional diseases of long standing, which originally sprang from corporeal maladies or were developed simultaneously with them.

§ 231.

The *intermittent diseases* deserve a special consideration, as well those that recur at certain periods—like the great number of intermittent fevers, and the apparently non-febrile affections that recur at intervals like intermittent fevers—as also those in which certain morbid states alternate at uncertain intervals with morbid states of a different kind.

§ 232.

These latter, *alternating* diseases, are also very numerous,[127] but all belong to the class of chronic dis-

---

[127] Two or three states may alternate with one another. Thus, for instance, in the case of double alternating diseases, certain pains may occur persistently in the legs, etc., immediately on the disappearance of a kind of ophthalmia, which latter again appears as soon as the pain in the limbs has gone off for the time—convulsions and spasms may alternate immediately with any other affection of the body or some part of it—in a case of threefold alternating states in a common indisposition, periods of

eases; they are generally a manifestation of developed psora alone, sometimes, but seldom, complicated with a syphilitic miasm, and therefore in the former case may be cured by antipsoric medicines; in the latter, however, in alternation with antisyphilitics as taught in my work on the *Chronic Diseases*.

§ 233.

The *typical intermittent diseases* are those where a morbid state of unvarying character returns at a tolerably fixed period, whilst the patient is apparently in good health, and takes its departure at an equally fixed period; this is observed in those apparently non-febrile morbid states that come and go in a periodical manner (at

---

apparent increase of health and unusual exaltation of the corporeal and mental powers (extravagant gaiety, extraordinary activity of the body, excess of comfortable feeling, inordinate appetite, etc.) may occur, after which, and quite unexpectedly, gloomy, melancholy humor, intolerable hypochondriacal derangement of the disposition, with disorder of several of the vital operations, the digestion, sleep, etc., appear, which again, and just as suddenly, give place to the habitual moderate ill-health; and so also several and very various alternating states. When the new state makes its appearance, there is often no perceptible trace of the former one. In other cases only slight traces of the former alternating state remain when the new one occurs; few of the symptoms of the first state remain on the appearance and during the continuance of the second. Sometimes the morbid alternating states are quite of opposite natures, as for instance, melancholy periodically alternating with gay insanity or frenzy.

certain times), as well as in those of a febrile character, to wit, the numerous varieties of intermittent fevers.

§ 234.

Those apparently non-febrile, typical, periodically recurring morbid states just alluded to observed in one single patient at a time (they do not usually appear sporadically or epidemically) always belong to the chronic diseases, mostly to those that are purely psoric, are but seldom complicated with syphilis, and are successfully treated by the same means; yet it is sometimes necessary to employ as an intermediate remedy a small dose of a potentized solution of cinchona bark, in order to extinguish completely their intermittent type.

§ 235.

With regard to the *intermittent fevers*,[128] that prevail sporadically or epidemically (not those endemically

---

[128] The pathology hitherto in vogue, which is still in the stage of irrational infancy, recognizes but one single *intermittent fever*, which it likewise termed *ague*, and admits of no varieties but such as are constituted by the different intervals at which the paroxysms recur, quotidian, tertian, quartan, etc. But there are much more important differences among them than what are marked by the periods of their recurrence; there are innumerable varieties of these fevers, some of which cannot even be denominated *ague*, as their fits consist solely of heat; others, again, are characterised by cold alone, with or without subsequent perspiration; yet others which exhibit general coldness of the surface, with a sensation of heat on the patient's part, or

located in marshy districts), we often find every paroxysm likewise composed of two opposite alternating

---

whilst the body feels externally hot, the patient feels cold;
others, again, in which one paroxysm consists entirely of a rigor
or simple chilliness, followed by an interval of health, while the
next consists of heat alone, followed or not by perspiration;
others, again, in which the heat comes first, and the cold stage
not till that is gone; others, again, wherein after a cold or hot
stage apyrexia ensues, and then perspiration comes on like a second fit, often many hours subsequently; others, again, in which
no perspiration at all comes on, and yet others in which the
whole attack consists of perspiration alone, without any cold or
hot stage, or in which the perspiration is only present during the
heat; and there are innumerable other differences, especially in
regard to the accessory symptoms, such as headache of a peculiar
kind, bad taste of the mouth, nausea, vomiting, diarrhœa, want of
or excessive thirst, peculiar pains in the body or limbs, disturbed
sleep, deliria, alterations of temper, spasms, etc., before, during
or after the cold stage, before, during or after the hot stage, before, during, or after the sweating stage, and countless other varieties.   All these are manifestly intermittent fevers of very different kinds, each of which, as might naturally be supposed, requires a special (homœopathic) treatment. It must be confessed
that they can almost all be suppressed (as is often done) by
enormous doses of bark and of its pharmaceutical preparation,
the *sulphate of quinine;* that is to say, their periodical recurrence (their typus) may be extinguished by it, but the patients
who suffered from intermittent fevers for which cinchona bark
is not suitable, as is the case with all those epidemic intermittent
fevers that traverse whole countries and even mountainous districts, are not restored to health by the extinction of the typus;
on the contrary, they now remain ill in another manner, and
worse, often much worse, than before; they are affected by
peculiar, chronic bark dyscrasias, and can scarcely be restored
to health even by a prolonged treatment by the true system of
medicine—and yet that is what is called *curing,* forsooth !

states (cold, heat—heat, cold), more frequently still of three (cold, heat, sweat). Therefore the remedy selected for them from the general class of proved (common, not antipsoric) medicines must either (and remedies of this sort are the surest) be able likewise to produce in the healthy body two (or all three) similar alternating states, or else must correspond by similarity of symptoms, in the most homœopathic manner possible, to the strongest, best marked, and most peculiar alternating state (either to the cold stage, or to the hot stage, or to the sweating stage, each with its accessory symptoms, according as the one or other alternating state is the strongest and most peculiar) ; but the symptoms of the patient's health during the intervals when he is free from fever must be the chief guide to the most appropriate homœopathic remedy.[129]

§ 236.

The most appropriate and efficacious time for administering the medicine in these cases is immediately or very soon after the termination of the paroxysm, as soon as the patient has in some degree recovered from its

---

[129] Dr. von Bönninghausen, who has rendered more services to our beneficent system of medicine than any other of my disciples, has best elucidated this subject, which demands so much care, and has facilitated the choice of the efficient remedy for the various epidemics of fever, in his work entitled *Versuch einer homöopathischen Therapie der Wechselfieber,* 1833, Münster bei Regensberg.

effects; it has then time to effect all the changes in the organism requisite for the restoration of health, without any great disturbance or violent commotion; whereas the action of a medicine, be it ever so specifically appropriate, if given immediately before the paroxysm, coincides with the natural recurrence of the disease and causes such a reaction in the organism, such a violent contention, that an attack of that nature produces at the very least a great loss of strength, if it do not endanger life.[130] But if the medicine be given immediately after the termination of the fit, that is to say, at the period when the apyretic interval has commenced and a long time before there are any preparations for the next paroxysm, then the vital force of the organism is in the best possible condition to allow itself to be quietly altered by the remedy, and thus restored to the healthy state.

§ 237.

But if the stage of apyrexia be very short, as happens in some very bad fevers, or if it be disturbed by some of the after sufferings of the previous paroxysm, the dose of the homœopathic medicine should be administered when the perspiration begins to abate, or the other subsequent phenomena of the expiring paroxysm begin to diminish.

---

[130] This is observed in the fatal cases, by no means rare, in which a moderate dose of opium given during the cold stage quickly deprived the patients of life.

§ 238.

Not infrequently, the suitable medicine has with a single dose destroyed several attacks and brought about the return of health, but in the majority of cases, another dose must be administered after each attack. Better still, however, when the character of the symptoms has not changed, doses of the same medicine given according to the newer discovery of repetition of doses (see note to § 270), may be given without difficulty by dynamizing each successive dose with 10-12 succussions of the vial containing the medicinal substance. Nevertheless, there are at times cases, though seldom, where the intermittent fever returns after several days' well being. This return of the same fever after a healthy interval is only possible when the noxious principle that first caused the fever, is still acting upon the convalescent, as is the case in marshy regions. Here a permanent restoration can often take place only by getting away from this causative factor, as is possible by seeking a mountainous retreat, if the cause was a marshy fever.

§ 239.

As almost every medicine causes in its pure action a special peculiar fever, and even a kind of intermittent fever with its alternating states, differing from all other fevers that are caused by other medicines, homœopathic remedies may be found in the extensive domain of medicines for all the numerous varieties of natural intermittent fevers and, for a great many of such fevers, even in the moderate collection of medicines already proved on the healthy individual.

§ 240.

But if the remedy found to be the homœopathic specific for a prevalent epidemic of intermittent fever do not effect a perfect cure in some one or other patient, if it be not the influence of a marshy district that prevents the cure, it must always be the psoric miasm in the background, in which case antipsoric medicines must be employed until complete relief is obtained.

§ 241.

Epidemics of intermittent fever in situations where none are endemic, are of the nature of chronic diseases, composed of single acute paroxysms; each single epidemy is of a peculiar, uniform character common to all the individuals attacked, and when this character is found in the totality of the symptoms common to all, it guides us to the discovery of the homœopathic (specific) remedy suitable for all the cases, which is almost universally serviceable in those patients who enjoyed tolerable health before the occurrence of the epidemy, that is to say, who were not chronic sufferers from developed psora.

§ 242.

If, however, in such an epidemic intermittent fever the first paroxysms have been left uncured, or if the patients have been weakened by improper allopathic treatment; then the inherent psora that exists, alas! in so many persons, although in a latent state, becomes developed, takes on the type of the intermittent fever, and to all appearances continues to play the part of the epidemic intermittent fever, so that the medicine, which would have been useful in the first paroxysms (rarely an antipsoric), is now no longer suitable and cannot be of any service. We have now to do with a psoric intermittent fever only, and this will generally be subdued by minute and rarely repeated doses of sulphur or hepar sulphuris in a high potency.

§ 243.

In those often very pernicious intermittent fevers which attack a single person, not residing in a marshy district, we must also *at first,* as in the case of acute diseases generally, which they resemble in respect to their psoric origin, employ for some days, to render what service it may, a homœopathic remedy selected for the special case from the other class of proved (not antipsoric) medicines; but if, notwithstanding this procedure the recovery is deferred, we know that we have to do with psora on the point of its development, and that in this case antipsoric medicines alone can effect a radical cure.

§ 244.

The intermittent fevers endemic in marshy districts and tracts of country frequently exposed to inundations, give a great deal of work to physicians of the old school, and yet a healthy man may in his youth become habituated even to marshy districts and remain in good health, provided he preserves a faultless regimen and his system is not lowered by want, fatigue or pernicious passions. The intermittent fevers endemic there would at the most only attack him on his first arrival; but one or two very small doses of a highly potentized solution of cinchona bark would, conjointly with the well-regulated mode of living just alluded to, speedily free him from the disease. But persons who, while taking sufficient corporeal exercise and pursuing a healthy system of intellectual occupations and bodily regimen, cannot be cured of marsh intermittent fever by one or a few of such small doses of cinchona—in such persons psora, striving to develop itself, always lies at the root of their malady, and their intermittent fever cannot be cured in the marshy district without antipsoric treatment.[131] It sometimes happens that when these patients exchange, without delay, the marshy district for one that is dry and mountainous, recovery apparently ensues (the fever leaves them) if

---

[131] Large, oft-repeated doses of cinchona bark, as also concentrated cinchonic remedies, such as the *sulphate of quinine,* have certainly the power of freeing such patients from the periodical fits of the marsh ague; but those thus deceived into the belief that they are cured remain diseased in another way, frequently with an incurable Quinin intoxication. (See § 276 note.)

they be not yet deeply sunk in disease, that is to say, if the psora was not completely developed in them and can consequently return to its latent state; but they will never regain perfect health without antipsoric treatment.

§ 245.

Having thus seen what attention should, in the homœopathic treatment, be paid to the chief varieties of diseases and to the peculiar circumstances connected with them, we now pass on to what we have to say respecting the remedies and the mode of employing them, together with the regimen to be observed during their use.

§ 246.

Every perceptibly progressive and strikingly increasing amelioration during treatment is a condition which, as long as it lasts, completely precludes every repetition of the administration of any medicine whatsoever, because all the good the medicine taken continues to effect is now hastening towards its completion. This is not infrequently the case in acute diseases, but in more chronic diseases, on the other hand, a single dose of an appropriately selected homœopathic remedy will at times complete even with but slowly progressive improvement and give the help which such a remedy in such a case can accomplish naturally within 40, 50, 60, 100 days. This is, however, but rarely the case; and besides, it must be a matter of great importance to the physician as well as to the patient that were it possible, this period should be diminished to one-half, one-quarter, and even still less, so that a much more rapid cure might be obtained. And this may be very happily effected, as recent and oft-repeated observations have taught me under the following conditions: firstly, if the medicine selected with the utmost care was perfectly homœopathic; secondly, if it is highly potentized, dissolved in water and given in proper small dose that experience has taught as the most suitable in definite intervals for the quickest accomplishment of the cure but with the precaution, *that the degree of every dose deviate somewhat from the preceding and following* in order that the vital principle which is to be altered to a similar medicinal disease be not aroused to untoward reactions and revolt as is always the case [133] with unmodified and especially rapidly repeated doses.

§ 247.

It is impractical to repeat the same unchanged dose of a remedy once, not to mention its frequent repetition

---

[133] What I said in the fifth edition of the *Organon*, in a long note to this paragraph in order to prevent these undesirable reactions of the vital energy, was all that the experience I then had justified. But during the last four or five years, however, all these difficulties are wholly solved by my new altered but perfected method. The same carefully selected medicine may now be given daily and for months, if necessary in this way, namely, after the lower degree of potency has been used for one or two weeks in the treatment of chronic disease, advance is made in the same way to higher degrees, (beginning according to the new dynamization method, taught herewith with the use of the lowest degrees).

(and at short intervals in order not to delay the cure). The vital principle does not accept such unchanged doses without resistance, that is, without other symptoms of the medicine to manifest themselves than those similar to the disease to be cured, because the former dose has already accomplished the expected change in the vital principle and a second dynamically wholly similar, unchanged dose of the same medicine no longer finds, therefore, the same conditions of the vital force. The patient may indeed be made sick in another way by receiving other such unchanged doses, even sicker than he was, for now only those symptoms of the given remedy remain active which were not homœopathic to the original disease, hence no step towards cure can follow, only a true aggravation of the condition of the patient. But if the succeeding dose is changed slightly every time, namely potentized somewhat higher (§§ 269-270) then the vital principle may be altered without difficulty by the same medicine (the sensation of natural disease diminishing) and thus the cure brought nearer.[133]

---

[133] We ought not even with the best chosen homœopathic medicine, for instance one pellet of the same potency that was beneficial at first, to let the patient have a second or third dose, taken dry. In the same way, if the medicine was dissolved in water and the first dose proved beneficial, a second or third and even smaller dose from the bottle *standing undisturbed,* even in intervals of a few days, would prove no longer beneficial, even though the original preparation had been potentized with ten succussions or as I suggested later with but two succussions in order to obviate this disadvantage and this according to above reasons. *But through modification of every dose in its dynamization degree,* as I herewith teach, there exists no offense, even if

§ 248.

For this purpose, we potentize anew the medicinal solution [134] (with perhaps 8, 10, 12 successions) from which we give the patient one or (increasingly) several teaspoonful doses, in long lasting diseases daily or every second day, in acute diseases every two to six hours and in very urgent cases every hour or oftener. Thus in

---

the doses be repeated more frequently, even if the medicine be ever so highly potentized with ever so many successions. It almost seems as if the best selected homœopathic remedy could best extract the morbid disorder from the vital force and in chronic diseases to extinguish the same only *if applied in several different forms.*

[134] Made in 40, 30, 20, 15 or 8 tablespoonfuls of water with the addition of some alcohol or a piece of charcoal in order to preserve it. If charcoal is used, it is suspended by means of a thread in the vial and is taken out when the vial is succussed. The solution of the medicinal globule (and it is rarely necessary to use more than one globule) of a thoroughly potentized medicine in a large quantity of water can be obviated by making a solution in only 7-8 tablespoonfuls of water and *after thorough succussion of the vial* take from it one tablespoonful and put it in a glass of water (containing about 7 to 8 spoonfuls), this *stirred thoroughly* and then give a dose to the patient. If he is unusually excited and sensitive, a teaspoonful of this solution may be put in a second glass of water, thoroughly stirred and teaspoonful doses or more be given. There are patients of so great sensitiveness that a third or fourth glass, similarly prepared, may be necessary. Each such prepared glass must be made fresh daily. The globule of the high potency is best crushed in a few grains of sugar of milk which the patient can put in the vial and be dissolved in the requisite quantity of water.

chronic diseases, every correctly chosen homœopathic medicine, even those whose action is of long duration, may be repeated daily for months with ever increasing success. If the solution is used up (in seven to fifteen days) it is necessary to add to the next solution of the same medicine if still indicated one or (though rarely) several pellets of a higher potency with which we continue so long as the patient experiences continued improvement without encountering one or another complaint that he never had before in his life. For if this happens, if the balance of the disease appears in a group of *altered* symptoms then *another, one more homœopathically related medicine must be chosen in place of the last and administered in the same repeated doses,* mindful, however, of modifying the solution of every dose with thorough vigorous succussions, thus changing its degree of potency and increasing it somewhat. On the other hand, should there appear during almost daily repetition of the well indicated homœopathic remedy, towards the end of the treatment of a chronic disease, *so-called* (§ 161) *homœopathic aggravations* by which the balance of the morbid symptoms seem to again increase somewhat (the medicinal disease, similar to the original, now alone persistently manifests itself). The doses in that case must then be reduced still further and repeated in longer intervals and possibly stopped several days, in order to see if the convalescence need no further medicinal aid. The apparent symptoms (Schein-Symptome) caused by the excess of the homœopathic medicine will soon disappear and leave undisturbed health in its wake. If only a small vial say a dram of dilute alcohol is used in the treatment, in which is contained and dissolved through succussion one globule of the medicine which is to be used by olfaction every two, three or four days, this also must be thoroughly succussed eight to ten times before each olfaction.

§ 249.

Every medicine prescribed for a case of disease which, in the course of its action, produces new and troublesome symptoms not appertaining to the disease to be cured, is not capable of effecting real improvement,[135] and cannot be considered as homœopathically selected; it must, therefore, either, if the aggravation be considerable, be first partially neutralized as soon as possible by an antidote before giving the next remedy chosen more accurately according to similarity of action; or if the

---

[135] As all experience shows that the dose of the specially suited homœopathic medicine can scarcely be prepared too small to effect perceptible amelioration in the disease for which it is appropriate (§§ 275-278), we should act injudiciously and hurtfully were we when no improvement, or some, though it be even slight, aggravation ensues, to repeat or even *increase the dose* of the same medicine, as is done in the old system, under the delusion that it was not efficacious on account of its small quantity (its too small dose). *Every aggravation by the production of new symptoms*—when nothing untoward has occurred in the mental or physical regimen —*invariably proves unsuitableness on the part of the medicine formerly given* in the case of disease before us, *but never indicates that the dose has been too weak.*

troublesome symptoms be not very violent, the next remedy must be given immediately, in order to take the place of the improperly selected one.[136]

§ 250.

When, to the observant practitioner who accurately investigates the state of the disease, it is evident, in urgent cases after the lapse of only six, eight or twelve hours that he has made a bad selection in the medicine last given, in that the patient's state is growing perceptibly, however slightly, worse from hour to hour, by the occurrence of new symptoms and sufferings, it is not only allowable for him, but it is his duty to remedy his mistake, by the selection and administration of a homœopathic medicine not merely tolerably suitable, but the most appropriate possible for the existing state of the disease (§ 167).

§ 251.

There are some medicines (e. g., ignatia, also bryonia and rhus, and sometimes belladonna) whose power of altering man's health consists chiefly in alternating actions—a kind of primary-action symptoms that are in

---

[136] The well informed and conscientiously careful physician will never be in a position to require an antidote in his practice if he will begin, as he should, to give the selected medicine in the smallest possible dose. A like minute dose of a better chosen remedy will re-establish order throughout.

part opposed to each other. Should the practitioner find, on prescribing one of these, selected on strict homœo-pathic principles, that no improvement follows, he will in most cases soon effect his object by giving (in acute dis-eases, even within a few hours) a fresh and equally small dose of the same medicine.[137]

§ 252.

But should we find, during the employment of the other medicines in chronic (psoric) diseases, that the best selected homœopathic (antipsoric) medicine in the suit-able (minutest) dose does not effect an improvement, this is a *sure* sign that the cause that keeps up the disease still persists, and that there is some circumstance in the mode of life of the patient or in the situation in which he is placed, that must be removed in order that a permanent cure may ensue.

§ 253.

Among the signs that, in all diseases, especially in such as are of an acute nature, inform us of a slight commencement of amelioration or aggravation that is not perceptible to every one, the state of mind and the whole demeanor of the patient are the most certain and in-structive. In the case of ever so slight an improvement

---

[137] As I have more particularly described in the introduction to "Ignatia" (in the first volume of the *Materia Medica Pura*).

we observe a greater degree of comfort, increased calmness and freedom of the mind, higher spirits—a kind of return of the natural state. In the case of ever so small a commencement of aggravation we have, on the contrary, the exact opposite of this: a constrained, helpless, pitiable state of the disposition, of the mind, of the whole demeanor, and of all gestures, postures and actions, which may be easily perceived on close observation, but cannot be described in words.[138]

§ 254.

The other new or increased symptoms, or, on the contrary, the diminution of the original ones without any addition of new ones, will soon dispel all doubts from the mind of the attentively observing and investigating

[138] The signs of improvement in the disposition and mind, however, may be expected only soon after the medicine has been taken when the dose has been *sufficiently minute* (*i. e.*, as small as possible), an unnecessarily larger dose of even the most suitable homoeopathic medicine acts too violently, and at first produces too great and too lasting a disturbance of the mind and disposition to allow us *soon* to perceive the improvement in them. I must here observe that this so essential rule is chiefly transgressed by presumptuous tyros in homoeopathy, and by physicians who are converted to homoeopathy from the ranks of the old school. From old prejudices these persons abhor the smallest doses of the lowest dilutions of medicine in such cases, and hence they fail to experience the great advantages and blessings of that mode of proceeding which a thousandfold experience has shown to be the most salutary; they cannot effect all that homoeopathy is capable of doing, and hence they have no claim to be considered its adherents.

practitioner with regard to the aggravation or amelioration; though there are among patients persons who are
either incapable of giving an account of this amelioration or aggravation, or are unwilling to confess it.

§ 255.

But even with such individuals we may convince ourselves on this point by going with them through all the
symptoms enumerated in our notes of the disease one by
one, and finding that they complain of no new unusual
symptoms in addition to these, and that none of the old
symptoms are worse. If this be the case, and if an improvement in the disposition and mind have already been
observed, the medicine must have effected positive diminution of the disease, or, if sufficient time have not yet
elapsed for this, it will soon effect it. If, now, the improvement delay too long in making its appearance, this
depends either on some error of conduct on the part of
the patient, or on other interfering circumstances.

§ 256.

On the other hand, if the patient mention the occurrence of some fresh accidents and symptoms of importance—signs that the medicine chosen has not been strictly
homœopathic—even though he should good-naturedly
assure us that he feels better, as is not infrequently the
case in phthisical patients with lung abscess, we must
not believe this assurance, but regard his state as aggravated as it will soon be perfectly apparent it is.

§ 257.

The true physician will take care to avoid making favorite remedies of medicines, the employment of which he has, by chance, perhaps found often useful, and which he has had opportunities of using with good effect. If he do so, some remedies of rarer use, which would have been more homœopathically suitable, consequently more serviceable, will often be neglected.

§ 258.

The true practitioner, moreover, will not in his practice with mistrustful weakness neglect the employment of those remedies that he may now and then have employed with bad effects, owing to an erroneous selection (from his own fault, therefore), or avoid them for other (false) reasons, as that they were unhomœopathic for the case of disease before him; he must bear in mind the truth, that of medicinal agents that one alone invariably deserves the preference in every case of disease which corresponds most accurately by similarity to the totality of the characteristic symptoms, and that no paltry prejudices should interfere with this serious choice.

§ 259.

Considering the minuteness of the doses necessary and proper in homœopathic treatment, we can easily understand that during the treatment everything must be removed from the *diet and regimen* which can have any medicinal action, in order that the small dose may not be overwhelmed and extinguished or disturbed by any foreign medicinal irritant.[139]

§ 260.

Hence the careful investigation into such obstacles to cure is so much the more necessary in the case of patients affected by chronic diseases, as their diseases are usually aggravated by such noxious influences and other disease-causing errors in the diet and regimen, which often pass unnoticed.[140]

---

[139] The softest tones of a distant flute that in the still midnight hours would inspire a tender heart with exalted feelings and dissolve it in religious ecstasy, are inaudible and powerless amid discordant cries and the noise of day.

[140] Coffee; fine Chinese and other herb teas; beer prepared with medicinal vegetable substances unsuitable for the patient's state; so-called fine liquors made with medicinal spices; all kinds of punch; spiced chocolate; odorous waters and perfumes of many kinds; strong-scented flowers in the apartment; tooth powders and essences and perfumed sachets compounded of drugs; highly spiced dishes and sauces; spiced cakes and ices; crude medicinal vegetables for soups; dishes of herbs, roots and stalks of plants possessing medicinal qualities; asparagus with long green tips, hops, and all vegetables possessing medicinal properties, celery, onions; old cheese, and meats that are in a state of decomposition, or that possess medicinal properties (as the flesh and fat of pork, ducks and geese, or veal that is too young and sour viands), ought just as certainly to be kept from patients as they should avoid all excesses in food, and in the use of sugar and salt, as also spirituous drinks, undiluted with water, heated rooms, woolen clothing next the skin, a sedentary life in close apartments, or the

§ 261.

The most appropriate regimen during the employment of medicine in chronic diseases consists in the removal of such obstacles to recovery, and in supplying where necessary the reverse: innocent moral and intellectual recreation, active exercise in the open air in almost all kinds of weather (daily walks, slight manual labor), suitable, nutritious, unmedicinal food and drink, etc.

§ 262.

In acute diseases, on the other hand—except in cases of mental alienation—the subtle, unerring internal sense of the awakened life-preserving faculty determines so clearly and precisely, that the physician only requires to counsel the friends and attendants to put no obstacles in the way of this voice of nature by refusing anything the

---

frequent indulgence in mere passive exercise (such as riding, driving or swinging), prolonged suckling, taking a long siesta in a recumbent posture in bed, sitting up long at night, uncleanliness, unnatural debauchery, enervation by reading obscene books, reading while lying down, Onanism or imperfect or suppressed intercourse in order to prevent conception, subjects of anger, grief, or vexation, a passion for play, over-exertion of mind or body, especially after meals, dwelling in marshy districts, damp rooms, penurious living, etc. All these things must be as far as possible avoided or removed, in order that the cure may not be obstructed or rendered impossible. Some of my disciples seem needlessly to increase the difficulties of the patient's dietary by forbidding the use of many more, tolerably indifferent things, which is not to be commended.

patient urgently desires in the way of food, or by trying
to persuade him to partake of anything injurious.

§ 263.

The desire of the patient affected by an acute disease
with regard to food and drink is certainly chiefly for
things that give palliative relief; they are, however, not
strictly speaking of a medicinal character, and merely
supply a sort of want. The slight hindrances that the
gratification of this desire, *within moderate bounds,* could
oppose to the radical removal of the disease[141] will be
amply counteracted and overcome by the power of the
homœopathically suited medicine and the vital force set
free by it, as also by the refreshment that follows from
taking what has been so ardently longed for. In like
manner, in acute diseases the temperature of the room
and the heat or coolness of the bed-coverings must also
be arranged entirely in conformity with the patient's
wish. He must be kept free from all over-exertion of
mind and exciting emotions.

§ 264.

The true physician must be provided with *genuine
medicines of unimpaired strength,* so that he may be able

---

[141] This is, however, rare. Thus, for instance, in pure inflammatory diseases, where aconite is so indispensable, whose action
would be destroyed by partaking of vegetable acids, the desire of
the patient is almost always for pure cold water only.

to rely upon their therapeutic powers; he must be able, *himself*, to judge of their genuineness.

§ 265.

It should be a matter of conscience with him to be thoroughly convinced in every case that the patient always takes the right medicine and therefore he must give the patient the correctly chosen medicine prepared, moreover, by himself.

§ 266.

Substances belonging to the animal and vegetable kingdom possess their medicinal qualities most perfectly in their raw state.[142]

---

[142] All crude animal and vegetable substances have a greater or less amount of medicinal power, and are capable of altering man's health, each in its own peculiar way. Those plants and animals used by the most enlightened nations as food have this advantage over all others, that they contain a larger amount of nutritious constituents; and they differ from the others in this that their medicinal powers in their raw state are either not very great in themselves, or are diminished by the culinary processes they are subjected to in cooking for domestic use, by the expression of the pernicious juice (like the cassava root of South America), by fermentation (of the rye-flour in the dough for making bread, sourcrout prepared without vinegar and pickled gherkins), by smoking and by the action of heat (in boiling, stewing, toasting, roasting, baking), whereby the medicinal parts of many of these substances are in part destroyed and dissipated. By the addition of salt (pickling) and vinegar (sauces, salads) animal and vege-

§ 267.

We gain possession of the powers of indigenous plants and of such as may be had in a fresh state in the most complete and certain manner by mixing their freshly expressed juice *immediately* with equal parts of spirits of wine of a strength sufficient to burn in a lamp. After this has stood a day and a night in a close stoppered bottle and deposited the fibrinous and albuminous matters, the clear superincumbent fluid is then to be decanted off for medicinal use.[143] All fermentation of the vegetable

---

table substances certainly lose much of their injurious medicinal qualities, but other disadvantages result from these additions.

But even those plants that possess most medicinal power lose that in part or completely by such processes. By perfect dessication all the roots of the various kinds of iris, of the horseradish, of the different species of arum and of the peonies lose almost all their medicinal virtue. The juice of the most virulent plants often becomes an inert, pitch-like mass, from the heat employed in preparing the ordinary extracts. By merely standing a long time, the expressed juice of the most deadly plants becomes quite powerless; even at a moderate atmospheric temperature it rapidly takes on the vinous fermentation (and thereby loses much of its medicinal power), and immediately thereafter the acetous and putrid fermentation, whereby it is deprived of all its peculiar medicinal properties; the fecula that is then deposited, if well washed, is quite innocuous, like ordinary starch. By the transudation that takes place when a number of green plants are laid one above the other, the greatest part of their medicinal properties is lost.

[143] Buchholz (*Taschenb. f. Scheidek. u. Apoth. a. d. J.*, 1815, Weimar, Abth. I, vi) assures his readers (and his reviewer in the *Leipziger Literaturzeitung*, 1816, No. 82, does not contradict him) that for this excellent mode of preparing medicines we have to thank the campaign in Russia, whence it was (in 1812)

juice will be at once checked by the spirits of wine mixed with it and rendered impossible for the future, and the entire medicinal power of the vegetable juice is thus retained (perfect and uninjured) *for ever* by keeping the preparation in well-corked bottles further protected with wax to prevent evaporation and excluded from the sun's light.[144]

---

imported into Germany. According to the noble practice of many Germans to be unjust towards their own countrymen, he conceals the fact that this discovery and those directions, which he quotes *in my very words* from the first edition of the *Organon of Rational Medicine*, § 230 and note, proceed from me, and that I *first* published them to the world two years before the Russian campaign (the *Organon* appeared in 1810). Some folks would rather assign the origin of a discovery to the deserts of Asia than to a German to whom the honor belongs. *O tempora! O mores!*

Alcohol has certainly been sometimes before this used for mixing with vegetable juices, *e. g.*, to preserve them some time before making extracts of them, but never with the view of administering them in this form.

[144] Although equal parts of alcohol and freshly expressed juice are usually the most suitable proportion for affecting the deposition of the fibrinous and albuminous matters, yet for plants that contain much thick mucus (*e. g.*, *Symphytum officinale, Viola tricolor*, etc.), or an excess of albumen (*e. g., Æthusa cynapium, Solanum nigrum*, etc.), a double proportion of alcohol is generally required for this object. Plants that are very deficient in juice, as *Oleander, Buxus, Taxus, Ledum, Sabina*, etc., must first be pounded up alone into a moist, fine mass and then stirred up with a double quantity of alcohol, in order that the juice may combine with it, and being thus extracted by the alcohol, may be pressed out; these latter may also when dried be brought with milk-sugar to the millionfold trituration, and then be further diluted and potentized (*v.* § 271).

§ 268.

The other exotic plants, barks, seeds and roots that cannot be obtained in the fresh state the sensible practitioner will never take in the pulverized form on trust, but will first convince himself of their genuineness in their crude, entire state before making any medicinal employment of them.[145]

---

[145] In order to preserve them in the form of powder, a precaution is requisite that has hitherto been usually neglected by druggists, and hence powders even of well-dried animal and vegetable substances could not be preserved uninjured even in well-corked bottles. The entire crude vegetable substances, though perfectly dry, yet contain, as an indispensable condition of the cohesion of their texture, a certain quantity of moisture, which does not indeed prevent the unpulverized drug from remaining in as dry a state as is requisite to preserve it from corruption, but which is quite too much for the finely pulverized state. The animal or vegetable substance which in its entire state was perfectly dry, furnishes therefore, when finely pulverized, a somewhat moist powder, which, without rapidly becoming spoilt and mouldy, can yet not be preserved in corked bottles if not previously freed from this superfluous moisture. This is best effected by spreading out the powder in a flat tin saucer with a raised edge, which floats in a vessel full of boiling water (*i. e.,* a water-bath), and, by means of stirring it about, drying it to such a degree that all the small atoms of it (no longer stick together in lumps, but) like dry, fine sand, are easily separated from each other, and are readily converted into dust. In this dry state the fine powders may be kept *forever* uninjured in well-corked and sealed bottles, in all their original complete medicinal power, *without ever being injured by mites or mould;* and they are best preserved when the bottles are kept protected from the daylight (in covered boxes, chests, cases). If not shut up in air-tight vessels, and not preserved from the

§ 269.

The homœopathic system of medicine develops for its special use, to a hitherto unheard-of degree, the inner medicinal powers of the crude substances by means of a process peculiar to it and which has hitherto never been tried, whereby only they all become immeasurably and penetratingly efficacious[146] and remedial, *even those that in the crude state give no evidence of the slightest medicinal power on the human body.*

This remarkable change in the qualities of natural bodies develops the latent, hitherto unperceived, as if slum-

---

access of the light of the sun and day, all animal and vegetable substances in time gradually lose their medicinal power more and more, even in the entire state, but still more in the form of powder.

[146] Long before this discovery of mine, experience had taught several changes which could be brought about in different natural substances by means of friction, for instance, warmth, heat, fire, development of odor in odorless bodies, magnetization of steel, and so forth. But all these properties produced by friction were related only to physical and inanimate things, whereas it is a law of nature according to which physiological and pathogenic changes take place in the body's condition by means of forces capable of changing the crude material of drugs, even in such as had never shown any medicinal properties. This is brought about by trituration and succussion, but under the condition of employing an indifferent vehicle in certain proportions. This wonderful physical and especially physiological and pathogenic law of nature had not been discovered before my time. No wonder then, that the present students of nature and physicians (so far unknowing) cannot have faith in the magical curative powers of the minute doses of medicines prepared according to homœopathic rules (dynamized).

bering[147] hidden, dynamic (§ 11) powers which influence the life principle, change the well-being of animal life.[148] This is effected by mechanical action upon their smallest particles by means of rubbing and shaking *and through the addition of an indifferent substance, dry or fluid, are*

---

[147] The same thing is seen in a bar of iron and steel where a slumbering trace of latent magnetic force cannot but be recognized in their interior. Both, after their completion by means of the forge stand upright, repulse the north pole of a magnetic needle with the lower end and attract the south pole, while the upper end shows itself as the south pole of the magnetic needle. But this is only a *latent* force; not even the finest iron particles can be drawn magnetically or held on either end of such a bar. Only after this bar of steel is *dynamized,* rubbing it with a dull file *in one direction,* will it become a true active powerful magnet, one able to attract iron and steel to itself and impart to another bar of steel by mere contact and even some distance away, magnetic power and this in a higher degree the more it has been rubbed. In the same way will triturating a medicinal substance and shaking of its solution (dynamization, potentiation) develop the medicinal powers hidden within and manifest them more and more or if one may say so, spiritualizes the material substance itself.

[148] On this account it refers only to the increase and stronger development of their power to cause changes in the *health* of animals and men if these natural substances in this improved state, are brought very near to the living sensitive fibre or come in contact with it (by means of intake or olfaction). Just as a magnetic bar especially if its magnetic force is increased (dynamized) can show magnetic power only in a needle of steel whose pole is near or touches it. The steel itself remains unchanged in the remaining chemical and physical properties and can bring about no changes in other metals (for instance, in brass), just as little as dynamized medicines can have any action upon *lifeless things.*

separated from each other. This process is called dynamizing, potentizing (development of medicinal power) and
the products are dynamizations[149] or potencies in different
degrees.

§ 270.

In order to best obtain this development of power, a
small part of the substance to be dynamized, say one grain,
is triturated for three hours with three times one hundred
grains sugar of milk according to the method described
below[150] up to the one-millionth part in powder
form. For reasons given below (b) one grain

---

[149] We hear daily how homœopathic medicinal potencies are
called *mere dilutions,* when they are the very opposite, *i. e.,* a
true opening up of the natural substances bringing to light and
revealing the hidden specific medicinal powers contained within
and brought forth by rubbing and shaking. The aid of a
chosen, unmedicinal medium of attenuation is but a *secondary
condition.*

Simple dilution, for instance, the solution of a grain of salt
will become water, the grain of salt will disappear in the dilution with much water and will never develop into medicinal salt
which by means of our well prepared dynamization, is raised to
most marvelous power.

[150] One-third of one hundred grains sugar of milk is put in a
glazed porcelain mortar, the bottom dulled previously by rubbing
it with fine, moist sand. *Upon this powder* is put one grain of
the powdered drug to be triturated (one drop of quicksilver,
petroleum, etc.). The sugar of milk used for dynamization
must be of that special pure quality that is crystallized on strings
and comes to us in the shape of long bars. For a moment the
medicine and powder are mixed with a porcelain spatula and
triturated rather strongly, six to seven minutes, with the pestle
rubbed dull, then the mass is scraped from the bottom of the

of this powder is dissolved in 500 drops of a mixture of one part of alcohol and four parts of distilled
water, of which *one drop* is put in a vial. To this are

---

mortar and from the pestle for three to four minutes, in order
to make it homogeneous. This is followed by triturating it in
the same way 6-7 minutes without adding anything more and
again scraping 3-4 minutes from what adhered to the mortar
and pestle. The second third of the sugar of milk is now
added, mixed with the spatula and again triturated 6-7 minutes,
followed by the scraping for 3-4 minutes and trituration without further addition for 6-7 minutes. The last third of sugar
of milk is then added, mixed with the spatula and triturated
as before 6-7 minutes with most careful scraping together. The
powder thus prepared is put in a vial, well corked, protected
from direct sunlight to which the name of the substance and
the designation of the first product marked $\overline{100}$ is given. In
order to raise this product to $\overline{10000}$, one grain of the powdered
$\overline{00}$ is mixed with the third part of 100 grains of powdered
sugar of milk and then proceed as before, but every third must
be carefully triturated twice thoroughly each time for 6-7 minutes and scraped together 3-4 minutes before the second and
last third of sugar of milk is added. After each third, the
same procedure is taken. When all is finished, the powder is
put in a well corked vial and labeled $\overline{10000}$. If now, one grain
of this last powder is taken in the same way, the 1/1,000,000, *i. e.*,
(1), each grain containing 1/1,000,000 the original substance.
Accordingly, such a trituration of the three degrees requires six
times six to seven minutes for triturating and six times 3-4
minutes for scraping, thus *one hour* for every degree. After
one hour such trituration of the first degree, each grain will
contain 1/000; of the second 1/10,000; and in the third 1/1,000,000
of the drug used.* Mortar, pestle and spatula must be cleaned

---

*These are the three degrees of the dry powder trituration,
which, if carried out correctly, will effect a good beginning for
the dynamization of the medicinal substance.

added 100 drops of pure alcohol[151] and given one hundred strong succussions with the hand against a hard but elastic body.[152] This is the medicine in the *first* degree of dynamization with which small sugar globules[153] may then be moistened[154] and quickly spread on blotting paper to dry and kept in a well-corked vial with the sign of (I) degree of potency. Only one[155] globule of this is taken

---

well before they are used for another medicine. Washed first with warm water and dried, both mortar and pestle, as well as spatula are then put in a kettle of boiling water for half an hour. Precaution might be used to *such an extent* as to put these utensils on a coal fire exposed to a glowing heat.

[151] The vial used for potentizing is filled two-thirds full.

[152] Perhaps on a leather bound book.

[153] They are prepared under supervision by the confectioner from starch and sugar and the small globules freed from fine dusty parts by passing them through a sieve. Then they are put through a strainer that will permit only 100 to pass through weighing one grain, the most serviceable size for the needs of a homœopathic physician.

[154] A small cylindrical vessel shaped like a thimble, made of glass, porcelain or silver, with a small opening at the bottom in which the globules are put to be medicated. They are moistened with some of the dynamized medicinal alcohol, stirred and poured out on blotting paper, in order to dry them quickly.

[155] According to first directions, one drop of the liquid of a lower potency was to be taken to 100 drops of alcohol for higher potentiation. This proportion of the medicine of attenuation to the medicine that is to be dynamized (100:1) was found altogether too limited to develop thoroughly and to a high degree the power of the medicine by means of a number

for further dynamization, put in a second new vial (with a drop of water in order to dissolve it) and then

---

of such succussions without specially using great force of which wearisome experiments have convinced me.

But if only one such globule be taken, of which 100 weigh one grain, and dynamize it with 100 drops of alcohol, the proportion of 1 to 50,000 and even greater will be had, for 500 such globules can hardly absorb one drop, for their saturation. With this disproportionate higher ratio between medicine and diluting medium *many* successive strokes of the vial filled two-thirds with alcohol can produce a much greater development of power. But with so small a diluting medium as 100 to 1 of the medicine, if many succussions by means of a powerful machine are forced into it, medicines are then developed which, especially in the higher degrees of dynamization, act almost immediately, but with furious, even dangerous, violence, especially in weakly patients, without having a lasting, mild reaction of the vital principle. But the method described by me, on the contrary, produces medicines of highest development of power and mildest action, which, however, if well chosen, touches all suffering parts curatively.* In acute fevers, the small doses of the lowest dynamization degrees of these thus perfected medicinal preparations, even of medicines of long continued action (for instance, belladonna) may be repeated in short intervals. In the treatment of chronic diseases, it is best to begin with the lowest degrees of dynamization and when necessary advance to higher, even more powerful but mildly acting degrees.

---

*In very rare cases, notwithstanding almost full recovery of health and with good vital strength, an old annoying local trouble continuing undisturbed it is wholly permitted and even *indispensably* necessary, to administer in increasing doses the homœopathic remedy that has proved itself efficacious but potentized to a very high degree by means of many succussions by hand. Such a local disease will often then disappear in a wonderful way.

with 100 drops of good alcohol and dynamized in the same way with 100 powerful succussions.

With this alcoholic medicinal fluid globules are again moistened, spread upon blotting paper and dried quickly, put into a well-stoppered vial and protected from heat and sun light and given the sign (II) of the second potency. And in this way the process is continued until the twenty-ninth is reached. Then with 100 drops of alcohol by means of 100 succussions, an alcoholic medicinal fluid is formed with which the thirtieth dynamization degree is given to properly moistened and dried sugar globules.

By means of this manipulation of crude drugs are produced preparations which only in this way reach the full capacity to forcibly influence the suffering parts of the sick organism. In this way, by means of a similar artificial morbid affection, the influence of the natural disease on the life principle present within is neutralized. By means of this mechanical procedure, provided it is carried out regularly according to the above teaching, a change is effected in the given drug, which in its crude state shows itself only as material, at times as unmedicinal material but by means of such higher and higher dynamization, it is changed and subtilized at last into spirit-like[156] medici-

---

[156] This assertion will not appear improbable, if one considers that by means of this method of dynamization (the preparations thus produced, I have found after many laborious experiments and counter-experiments, to be the most powerful and at the same time mildest in action, i. e., as the most perfected) the material part of the medicine is lessened with each degree of dynamization 50,000 times and yet incredibly increased in power, so that the further dynamization of 125 and 18 ciphers

nal power, which, indeed, *in itself* does not fall within our
senses but for which the medicinally prepared globule,
dry, but more so when dissolved in water, becomes *the
carrier,* and in this condition, manifests the healing power
of this invisible force in the sick body.

§ 271.

If the physician prepares his homœopathic medicines
himself, as he should reasonably do in order to save
men from sickness,[157] he may use the fresh plant itself,
as but little of the crude article is required, if he does not
need the expressed juice perhaps for purposes of healing.
He takes a few grains in a mortar and with 100 grains
sugar of milk three distinct times brings them to the one-

---

reaches only the third degree of dynamization. The thirtieth
thus progressively prepared would give a fraction almost impossible to be expressed in numbers. It becomes uncommonly
evident that the material part by means of such dynamization
(development of its true, inner medicinal essence) will ultimately
dissolve into its individual spirit-like, (conceptual) essence. In
its crude state therefore, it may be considered to consist really
only of this undeveloped conceptual essence.

[157] Until the State, in the future, after having attained insight
into the indispensability of perfectly prepared homœopathic
medicines, will have them manufactured by a competent im-
partial person, in order to give them free of charge to homœopathic physicians trained in homœopathic hospitals, who have
been examined theoretically and practically, and thus legally
qualified. The physician may then become convinced of these
divine tools for purposes of healing, but also to give them free
of charge to his patients—rich and poor.

millionth trituration (§ 270) before further potentizing of
a small portion of this by means of shaking is undertaken,
a procedure to be observed also with the rest of crude
drugs of either dry or oily nature.

§ 272.

Such a globule,[158] placed dry upon the tongue, is one of
the smallest doses for a moderate recent case of illness.
Here but few nerves are touched by the medicine. A similar globule, crushed with some sugar of milk and dissolved
in a good deal of water (§ 247) and stirred well before
every administration will produce a far more powerful
medicine for the use of several days. Every dose, no matter how minute, touches, on the contrary, many nerves.

§ 273.

In no case under treatment is it necessary and *therefore
not permissible* to administer to a patient more than *one
single, simple medicinal* substance at one time. It is inconceivable how the slightest doubt could exist as to whether
it was more consistent with nature and more rational to
prescribe a *single, simple*[159] medicine at one time in a dis-

---

[158] These globules (§ 270) retain their medicinal virtue for
many years, if protected against sunlight and heat.

[159] Two substances, opposite to each other, united into neutral
Natrum and middle salts by chemical affinity in unchangeable
proportions, as well as sulphuretted metals found in the earth
and those produced by technical art in constant combining pro-

ease or a mixture of several differently acting drugs. It is absolutely not allowed in homœopathy, the one true, simple and natural art of healing, to give the patient *at one time* two different medicinal substances.

§ 274.

As the true physician finds in simple medicines, administered singly and uncombined, all that he can possibly desire (artificial disease-forces which are able by homœopathic power completely to overpower, extinguish, and permanently cure natural diseases), he will, mindful of the wise maxim that "it is wrong to attempt to employ complex means when simple means suffice," never think of giving as a remedy any but a single, simple medicinal substance; for these reasons also, because even though the simple medicines were *thoroughly proved* with respect to their pure peculiar effects on the unimpaired healthy

---

portions of sulphur and alkaline salts and earths, for instance (natrum sulph. and calcarea sulph.) as well as those ethers produced by distillation of alcohol and acids may together with phosphorus be considered as *simple* medicinal substances by the homœopathic physician and used for patients. On the other hand, those extracts obtained by means of acids of the so-called alkaloids of plants, are exposed to great variety in their preparation (for instance, chinin, strychnine, morphine), and can, therefore, not be accepted by the homœopathic physician as simple medicines, always the same, especially as he possesses, in the plants themselves, in their natural state (Peruvian bark, nux vomica, opium) every quality necessary for healing. Moreover, the alkaloids are not the only constituents of the plants.

state of man, it is yet impossible to foresee *how* two and more medicinal substances might, when compounded, hinder and alter each other's actions on the human body; and because, on the other hand, a simple medicinal substance when used in diseases, the totality of whose symptoms is accurately known, renders efficient aid by itself alone, if it be homœopathically selected; and supposing the worst case to happen, that it was not chosen in strict conformity to similarity of symptoms, and therefore does no good, it is yet so far useful that it promotes our knowledge of therapeutic agents, because, by the new symptoms excited by it in such a case, those symptoms which this medicinal substance had already shown in experiments, on the healthy human body are confirmed, an advantage that is lost by the employment of all compound remedies.[160]

§ 275.

The suitableness of a medicine for any given case of disease does not depend on its accurate homœopathic selection alone, but likewise on the proper size, or rather smallness, of the dose. If we give *too strong a dose* of a medicine which may have been even quite homœopathically chosen for the morbid state before us, it must, notwith-

---

[160] When the rational physician has chosen the perfectly homœopathic medicine for the well-considered case of disease and administered it internally, he will leave to irrational allopathic routine the practice of giving drinks or fomentations of different plants, of injecting medicated glysters and of rubbing in this or the other ointment.

standing the inherent beneficial character of its nature, prove injurious by its mere magnitude, and by the unnecessary, too strong impression which, by virtue of its homœopathic similarity of action, it makes upon the vital force which it attacks and, through the vital force, upon those parts of the organism which are the most sensitive, and are already most affected by the natural disease.

§ 276.

For this reason, a medicine, even though it may be homœopathically suited to the case of disease, does harm in every dose that is too large, and in strong doses it does more harm the greater its homœopathicity and the higher the potency[161] selected, and it does much more injury than any equally large dose of a medicine that is unhomœopathic and in no respect adapted to the morbid state (allopathic).

Too large doses of an accurately chosen homœopathic medicine, and especially when frequently repeated, bring about much trouble as a rule. They put the patient not seldom in danger of life or make his disease almost incurable. They do indeed extinguish the natural disease so

---

[161] The praise bestowed of late years by some few homœopathists on the larger doses is owing to this, either that they chose low dynamizations of the medicine to be administered (as I myself used to do twenty years ago, from not knowing any better), or that the medicines selected were not homœopathic and imperfectly prepared by their manufacturers.

far as the sensation of the life principle is concerned and the patient no longer suffers from the original disease from the moment the too strong dose of the homœopathic medicine acted upon him but he is in consequence more ill with the similar but more violent medicinal *disease which* is most difficult to destroy.[162]

§ 277.

For the same reason, and because a medicine, provided the dose of it was sufficiently small, is all the more salutary and almost marvellously efficacious the more accurately homœopathic its selection has been, a medicine

---

[162]Thus, the continuous use of aggressive allopathic large doses of mercurials against syphilis develops almost incurable mercurial maladies, when yet one or several doses of a mild but active mercurial preparation would certainly have radically cured in a few days the whole venereal disease, together with the chancre, provided it had not been destroyed by external measures (as is always done by allopathy). In the same way, the allopath gives Peruvian bark and quinine in intermittent fever daily in very large doses, where they are correctly indicated and where one very small dose of a highly potentized China would unfailingly help (in marsh intermittents and even in persons who were not affected by any evident psoric disease). A chronic China malady (coupled at the same time with the development of psora) is produced, which, if it does not gradually kill the patient by damaging the internal important vital organs, especially spleen and liver, will put him, nevertheless, suffering for years in a sad state of health. A homœopathic antidote for such a misfortune produced by abuse of large doses of homœopathic remedies is hardly conceivable.

whose selection has been accurately homœopathic must be all the more salutary the more its dose is reduced to the degree of minuteness appropriate for a gentle remedial effect.

§ 278.

Here the question arises, what is this most suitable degree of minuteness for sure and gentle remedial effect; how small, in other words, must be the dose of each individual medicine, homœopathically selected for a case of disease, to effect the best cure? To solve this problem, and to determine for every particular medicine, what dose of it will suffice for homœopathic therapeutic purposes and yet be so minute that the gentlest and most rapid cure may be thereby obtained—to solve this problem is, as may easily be conceived, not the work of theoretical speculation; not by fine-spun reasoning, not by specious sophistry, can we expect to obtain the solution of this problem. It is just as impossible as to tabulate in advance all imaginable cases. Pure experiment, careful observation of the sensitiveness of each patient, and accurate experience can alone determine this *in each individual case,* and it were absurd to adduce the large doses of unsuitable (*allopathic*) medicines of the old system, which do not touch the diseased side of the organism homœopathically, but only attack the parts unaffected by the disease, in opposition to what pure experience pronounces respecting the smallness of the doses required for homœopathic cures.

20

§ 279.

This pure experience shows UNIVERSALLY, that if the disease do not manifestly depend on a considerable deterioration of an important viscus (even though it belong to the chronic and complicated diseases), and if during the treatment all other alien medicinal influences are kept away from the patient, *the dose of the homœo-pathically selected and highly potentized remedy* for the beginning of treatment of an important, especially chronic disease can never be prepared so small that it shall not be stronger than the natural disease and shall not be able to overpower it, at least in part and extinguish it from the sensation of the principle of life and thus make a beginning of a cure.

§ 280.

The dose of the medicine that continues serviceable without producing new troublesome symptoms is to be continued while *gradually ascending,* so long as the patient *with general improvement,* begins to feel in a mild degree the return of one or several old original complaints. This indicates an approaching cure through a gradual ascending of the moderate doses modified each time by succussion (§ 247). It indicates that the vital principle no longer needs to be affected by the similar medicinal disease in order to lose the sensation of the natural disease (§ 148). It indicates that the life principle now free from the natural disease begins to suffer only something of the medicinal disease hitherto known as *homœopathic aggravation.*

§ 281.

In order to be convinced of this, the patient is left without any medicine for eight, ten or fifteen days, meanwhile giving him only some powders of sugar of milk. If the few last complaints are due to the medicine simulating the former original disease symptoms, then these complaints will disappear in a few days or hours. If during these days without medicine, while continuing good hygienic regulations nothing more of the original disease is seen, he is probably cured. But if in the later days traces of the former morbid symptoms should show themselves, they are remnants of the original disease not wholly extinguished, which must be treated with renewed higher potencies of the remedy as directed before. If a cure is to follow, the first small doses must likewise be again gradually raised higher, but less and more slowly in patients where considerable irritability is evident than in those of less susceptibility, where the advance to higher dosage may be more rapid. There are patients whose impressionability compared to that of the unsusceptible ones is like the ratio as 1000 to 1.

§ 282.

It would be a certain sign that the doses were altogether too large, if during treatment, especially in chronic diseases, the first dose should bring forth a so-called *homœopathic aggravation,* that is, a marked increase of the original morbid symptoms first discovered and in the same way every repeated dose (§ 247) however modified somewhat by shaking before its administration (*i. e.,* more highly dynamized).[163]

---

[163] The rule to commence the homœopathic treatment of chronic diseases with the smallest possible doses and only gradually to augment them is subject to a notable exception in the treatment of the three great miasms while they still effloresce on the skin, *i. e.,* recently erupted *itch,* the untouched *chancre* (on the sexual organs, labia, mouth or lips, and so forth), and the *figwarts.* These not only tolerate, but indeed require, from the very beginning large doses of their specific remedies of ever higher and higher degrees of dynamization daily (possibly also several times daily). If this course be pursued, there is no danger to be feared as is the case in the treatment of diseases hidden within, that the excessive dose while it extinguishes the disease, initiates and by continued usage possibly produces a chronic medicinal disease. During external manifestations of these three miasms this is not the case; for from the daily progress of their treatment it can be observed and judged to what degree the large dose withdraws the sensation of the disease from the vital principle day by day; for none of these three can be cured without giving the physician the conviction through their disappearance that there is no longer any further need of these medicines.

Since diseases in general are but dynamic attacks upon the life principle and nothing material—no *materia peccans*—as their basis (as the old school in its delusion has fabulated for a thousand years and treated the sick accordingly to their ruin) there is also in these cases nothing material to take away, nothing to smear away, to burn or tie or cut away, without making the patient endlessly sicker and more incurable (Chron. Dis. Part 1), than he was before local treatment of these three miasms was instituted. The dynamic, inimical principle exerting its influence upon the vital energy is the essence of these external signs of the inner malignant miasms that can be extinguished

§ 283.

In order to work wholly according to nature, the true healing artist will prescribe the accurately chosen homœopathic medicine most suitable in all respects in so small a dose on account of this alone. For should he be misled by human weakness to employ an unsuitable medicine, the disadvantage of its wrong relation to the disease would be so small that the patient could through his own vital powers and by means of early opposition (§ 249) of the correctly chosen remedy according to symptom similarity (and this also in the smallest dose) rapidly extinguish and repair it.

§ 284.

Besides the tongue, mouth and stomach, which are most commonly affected by the administration of medicine, the nose and respiratory organs are receptive

---

solely by the action of a homœopathic medicine upon the vital principle which affects it in a similar but stronger manner and thus extracts the sensation of internal and external spirit-like (conceptual) disease enemy in such a way that it no longer exists for the life principle (for the organism) and thus releases the patient of his illness and he is cured.

Experience, however, teaches that the itch, plus its external manifestations, as well as the chancre, together with the inner venereal miasm, can and must be cured only by means of specific medicines taken internally. But the figwarts, if they have existed for some time without treatment, have need for their perfect cure, the external application of their specific medicines as well as their internal use at the same time.

of the action of medicines in fluid form by means of
olfaction and inhalation through the mouth. But the
whole remaining skin of the body clothed with epidermis,
is adapted to the action of medicinal solutions, especially
if the inunction is connected with simultaneous internal
administration.[164]

§ 285.

In this way, the cure of very old diseases may be
furthered by the physician applying externally, rubbing
it in the back, arms, extremities, the same medicine he

---

[164] The power of medicines acting upon the infant through the
milk of the mother or wet nurse is wonderfully helpful. Every
disease in a child yields to the rightly chosen homœopathic
medicines given in moderate doses to the nursing mother and
so administered, is more easily and certainly utilized by these
new world-citizens than is possible in later years. Since most
infants usually have imparted to them psora through the milk
of the nurse, if they do not already possess it through heredity
from the mother, they may be at the same time protected
antipsorically by means of the milk of the nurse rendered
medicinally in this manner. But the case of mothers in their
(first) pregnancy by means of a mild antipsoric treatment,
especially with sulphur dynamizations prepared according to the
directions in this edition (§ 270), is indispensable in order to
destroy the psora—that producer of most chronic diseases—
which is given them hereditarily; destroy it both within themselves and in the fœtus, thereby protecting posterity in advance.
This is true of pregnant women thus treated; they have given
birth to children usually more healthy and stronger, to the
astonishment of everybody. A new confirmation of the great
truth of the psora theory discovered by me.

gives internally and which showed itself curatively. In doing so, he must avoid parts subject to pain or spasm or skin eruption.[165]

---

[165] From this fact may be explained those marvelous cures, however infrequent, where chronic deformed patients, whose skin nevertheless was *sound and clean,* were cured quickly and permanently after a few baths whose medicinal constituents (by chance) were homœopathically related. On the other hand, the mineral baths *very often* brought on increased injury with patients, whose eruptions on the skin were suppressed. After a brief period of well-being, the life principle allowed the inner, uncured malady to appear elsewhere, more important for life and health.

At times, instead, the ocular nerve would become paralyzed and produce amaurosis, sometimes the crystaline lens would become clouded, hearing lost, mania or suffocating asthma would follow or an apoplexy would end the sufferings of the deluded patient.

A fundamental principle of the homœopathic physician (which distinguishes him from every physician of all older schools) is this, that he never employs for any patient a medicine, whose effects on the healthy human has not previously been carefully proven and thus made known to him (§§ 20, 21). To prescribe for the sick on mere conjecture of some possible usefulness for some similar disease or from hearsay "that a remedy has helped in such and such a disease"—such conscienceless venture the philanthropic homœopathist will leave to the allopath. A genuine physician and practitioner of our art will therefore *never* send the sick to any of the numerous mineral baths, because almost all are unknown so far as their accurate, positive effects on the healthy human organism is concerned, and when misused, must be counted among the most violent and dangerous drugs. In this way, out of a thousand sent to the most celebrated of these baths by ignorant physicians allopathically uncured and blindly sent there perhaps one or two are cured by

§ 286.

The dynamic force of mineral magnets, electricity and galvanism act no less powerfully upon our life principle and they are not less homœopathic than the properly so-called medicines which neutralize disease by taking them through the mouth, or by rubbing them on the skin or by olfaction. There may be diseases, especially diseases of sensibility and irritability, abnormal sensations, and involuntary muscular movements which may be cured by those means. But the more certain way of applying the last two as well as that of the so-called electro-magnetic machine lies still very much in the dark to make homœopathic use of them. So far both electricity and Galvanism have been used only for palliation to the great damage of the sick. The positive, pure action of both upon the healthy human body have until the present time been but little tested.

---

chance more often return only *apparently* cured and the miracle is proclaimed aloud. Hundreds, meanwhile sneak quietly away, more or less worse and the rest remain to prepare themselves for their eternal resting place, a fact that is verified by the presence of numerous well-filled graveyards surrounding the most celebrated of these spas.*

---

*A true homœopathic physician, one who never acts without correct fundamental principles, never gambles with the life of the sick entrusted to him as in a lottery where the winner is in the ratio of 1 to 500 or 1000 (blanks here consisting of aggravation or death), will never expose any one of his patients to such danger and send him for good luck to a mineral bath, as is done so frequently by allopaths in order to get rid of the sick in an acceptable manner spoiled by him or others.

§ 287.

The powers of the magnet for healing purposes can be employed with more certainty according to the positive effects detailed in the *Materia Medica Pura* under north and south pole of a powerful magnetic bar. Though both poles are alike powerful, they nevertheless oppose each other in the manner of their respective action. The doses may be modified by the length of time of contact with one or the other pole, according as the symptoms of either north or south pole are indicated. As antidote to a too violent action the application of a plate of polished zinc will suffice.

§ 288.

I find it yet necessary to allude here to *animal magnetism,* as it is termed, or rather *Mesmerism* (as it should be called in deference to Mesmer, its first founder) which differs so much in its nature from all other therapeutic agents. This curative force, often so stupidly denied and disdained for a century, acts in different ways. It is a marvelous, priceless gift of God to mankind by means of which the strong will of a well intentioned person upon a sick one by contact and even without this and even at some distance, can bring the vital energy of the healthy mesmeriser endowed with this power into another person dynamically (just as one of the poles of a powerful magnetic rod upon a bar of steel).

It acts in part by replacing in the sick whose vital force within the organism is deficient here and there, in part also in other parts where the vital force has accumulated too much and keeps up irritating nervous disorders it turns it aside, diminishes and distributes it equally and in general extinguishes the morbid condition of the life principle of the patient and substitutes in its place the normal of the mesmerist acting powerfully upon him, for instance, old ulcers, amaurosis, paralysis of single organs and so forth. Many rapid apparent cures performed in all ages, by mesmerizers endowed with great natural power, belong to this class. The effect of communicated human power upon the whole human organism was most brilliantly shown, in the resuscitation of persons who had lain some time apparently dead, by the most powerful sympathetic will of a man in full vigor of vital energy,[166] and of this kind of resurrection history records many undeniable examples.

If the mesmerizing person of either sex capable at the same time of a good-natured enthusiasm (even its degeneration into bigotry, fanaticism, mysticism or philanthropic dreaming) will be empowered all the more with this philanthropic self-sacrificing performance to direct exclusively the power of his commanding good

---

[166] Especially of one of such persons, of whom there are not many, who, along with great kindness of disposition and perfect bodily powers, possesses but *a very moderate desire for sexual intercourse,* which it would give him very little trouble wholly to suppress, in whom, consequently, all the fine vital spirits that would otherwise be employed in the preparation of the semen, are ready to be communicated to others, by touching them and powerfully exerting the will. Some powerful mesmerisers, with whom I have become acquainted, had *all* this peculiar character.

will to the recipient requiring his help and at the same time to concentrate these, he may at times perform apparent miracles.

§ 289.

All the above-mentioned methods of practising mesmerism depend upon an influx of more or less vital force into the patient, and hence are termed positive mesmerism.[167] An opposite mode of employing mesmerism, however, as it produces just the contrary effect, deserves to be termed negative mesmerism. To this belong the passes which are used to rouse from the somnambulic sleep, as also all the manual processes known by the names of *soothing and ventilating*. This *discharge* by means of negative mesmerism of the vital force accumulated to excess in individual parts of the system of undebilitated persons is most surely and simply performed by making a very rapid motion of the flat extended hand, held parallel to, and about an inch distant from the body,

---

[167] When I here speak of the decided and certain curative power of positive mesmerism, I most assuredly do not mean that abuse of it, where, by repeated passes of this kind, continued for half an hour or a whole hour at a time, and, even day after day, performed on weak, nervous patients, that monstrous revolution of the whole human system is effected which is termed somnambulism, wherein the human being is ravished from the world of sense and seems to belong more to the world of spirits—a highly unnatural and dangerous state, by means of which it has not infrequently been attempted to cure chronic diseases.

from the top of the head to the tips of the toes.[168] The more rapidly this pass is made, so much the more effectually will the discharge be effected. Thus, for instance, in the case where a previously healthy woman,[169] from the sudden suppression of her catamenia by a violent mental shock, lies to all appearance dead, the vital force which is probably accumulated in the præcordial region, will, by such a rapid negative pass, be discharged and its equilibrium throughout the whole organism restored, so that the resuscitation generally follows immediately.[170] In like manner, a gentle, less rapid, negative pass diminishes the excessive restlessness and sleeplessness accompanied with anxiety sometimes produced in very irritable persons by a too powerful positive pass, etc.

---

[168] It is a well known rule that a person who is either to be positively or negatively mesmerised, should not wear silk on any part of the body.

[169] Hence a negative pass, especially if it be very rapid, is extremely injurious to a delicate person affected with a chronic ailment and deficient in vital force.

[170] A strong country lad, ten years of age, received in the morning, on account of slight indisposition, from a professed female mesmeriser, several very powerful passes with the points of both thumbs, from the pit of the stomach along the lower edge of the ribs, and he instantly grew deathly pale, and fell into such a state of unconsciousness and immobility that no effort could arouse him, and he was almost given up for dead. I made his eldest brother give him a very rapid negative pass from the crown of the head over the body to the feet, and in one instant he recovered his consciousness and became lively and well.

§ 290.

Here belongs also the so-called massage of a vigorous good-natured person given to a chronic invalid, who, though cured, still suffers from loss of flesh, weakness of digestion and lack of sleep due to slow convalescence. The muscles of the limbs, breast and back, separately grasped and moderately pressed and kneaded arouse the life principle to reach and restore the tone of the muscles and blood and lymph vessels. The mesmeric influence of this procedure is the chief feature and it must not be used to excess in patients still hypersensitive.

§ 291.

Baths of pure water prove themselves partly palliative, partly as homœopathic serviceable aids in restoring health in acute diseases as well as in convalescence of cured chronic patients with proper consideration of the conditions of the convalescent and the temperature of the bath, its duration and repetition. But even if well applied, they bring only physically beneficial changes in the sick body, in themselves they are no true medicine. The lukewarm baths at 25 to 27° R. serve to arouse the slumbering sensibility of fibre in the apparent dead (frozen, drowned, suffocated) which benumbed the sensation of the nerves. Though only palliative, still they often prove themselves sufficiently active, especially when given in conjunction with coffee and rubbing with the hands. They may give homœopathic aid in cases where the irritability is very unevenly distributed and accumulated too unevenly in some organs as is the case in certain hysteric spasms and infantile convulsions. In the same way, cold baths 10 to 6° R. in persons cured medically of chronic diseases and with deficiency of vital heat, act as a homœopathic aid. By *instantaneous* and later with *repeated* immersions they act as a palliative restorative of the tone of the exhausted fibre. For this purpose, such baths are to be used for more than momentary duration, rather for minutes and of gradually lowered temperature, they are a palliative, which, since it acts only physically has no connection with the disadvantage of a reverse action to be feared afterwards, as takes place with dynamic medicinal palliatives.